"One of the greatest sources of stress for parents is feeling unable to help their kids with stress. Thankfully, two leading experts have written an informative, practical book that will make it easier to understand—and support—children and teens with anxiety and depression."

—**Adam Grant**, *New York Times* bestselling author
of *Think Again* and *Option B*

"In this timely masterpiece of a book, Khanna and Kendall give parents the tools to prevent, address, and overcome childhood anxiety. Building on decades of scientific evidence, and translating all of it into clear, practical steps that parents can use right away. It's the closest thing to having the greatest minds in the field of childhood anxiety by your side, coaching you every step of the way!"

—**Eli R. Lebowitz, PhD**, associate professor at the Yale
Child Study Center, and author of *Breaking Free of Child
Anxiety and OCD*

"This valuable book provides excellent advice to help anxious kids (and anxious parents) learn important skills to manage their anxiety and thrive, even in a period of uncertainty. It is written in a clear, accessible way, and provides a concrete four-step program with 'conversation starters' to engage and motivate children and teens to participate. This book will be useful not only for parents and caregivers, but also for school counselors and therapists."

—**Judith S. Beck, PhD**, president of the nonprofit
Beck Institute for Cognitive Behavior Therapy, and
author of *Cognitive Behavior Therapy*

T0000251

"Khanna and Kendall delivered what parents (and policymakers) have long needed—pragmatic, evidence-based guidance on how to instill resilience in our kids and contribute to the betterment of our nation's public health. As we all witnessed throughout the pandemic, *The Resilience Recipe* is exactly what parents need to counter the growing mental health toll on our children."

> —**Aneesh Chopra**, former US Chief Technology Officer (2009-2012), and author of *Innovative State*

"Our children are being overwhelmed by the challenges of the modern world, but you can help. Resilience is a skill that children can learn step by step, and like a coach who does not expect mastery on day one, when you understand what resilience is and where it comes from you can gain the patience and wisdom to support that learning process. Mixing methods, concepts, and findings from all of the waves and eras of the cognitive behavioral tradition, this gentle and wise volume will help your child learn to feel their feelings, manage their judgments, and choose actions that produce positive outcomes."

> —**Steven C. Hayes, PhD**, Nevada Foundation Professor in the department of psychology at the University of Nevada, Reno; and originator and codeveloper of acceptance and commitment therapy (ACT)

"Every parent or caregiver with a child who worries or experiences anxiety needs to read *The Resilience Recipe* and implement its science-based strategies. Based on years of practice and research, internationally renowned experts Khanna and Kendall provide clear and specific guidance on HOW to relieve anxieties and bounce back. Their user-friendly tips make this a particularly valuable book for parents. Readers will appreciate the 'key takeaways' and 'conversation starters.'"

> —**Mary K. Alvord, PhD**, psychologist, and coauthor of *Resilience Builder Program for Children and Adolescents* and *Conquer Negative Thinking for Teens*

The
Resilience
Recipe

A Parent's Guide to
Raising Fearless Kids
in the Age of Anxiety

MUNIYA S. KHANNA, PHD

PHILIP C. KENDALL, PHD, ABPP

New Harbinger Publications, Inc.

Publisher's Note

This publication is designed to provide accurate and authoritative information in regard to the subject matter covered. It is sold with the understanding that the publisher is not engaged in rendering psychological, financial, legal, or other professional services. If expert assistance or counseling is needed, the services of a competent professional should be sought.

Distributed in Canada by Raincoast Books

NEW HARBINGER PUBLICATIONS is a registered trademark of New Harbinger Publications, Inc.

Copyright © 2021 by Muniya S. Khanna and Philip C. Kendall
New Harbinger Publications, Inc.
5674 Shattuck Avenue
Oakland, CA 94609
www.newharbinger.com

Cover design by Sara Christian

Acquired by Tesilya Hanauer

Edited by Kristi Hein

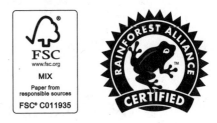

FSC
www.fsc.org
MIX
Paper from responsible sources
FSC® C011935

Library of Congress Cataloging-in-Publication Data

Names: Khanna, Muniya S., author. | Kendall, Philip C., author.
Title: The resilience recipe : a parent's guide to raising fearless kids in the age of anxiety / Muniya S. Khanna, Ph.D., Philip C. Kendall, Ph.D., ABPP.
Description: Oakland, CA : New Harbinger Publications, Inc., [2021] | Includes bibliographical references.
Identifiers: LCCN 2021021229 | ISBN 9781684036967 (trade paperback)
Subjects: LCSH: Resilience (Personality trait) in children. | Anxiety in children.
Classification: LCC BF723.R46 K43 2021 | DDC 155.4/1824--dc23
LC record available at https://lccn.loc.gov/2021021229

Printed in the United States of America

23   22   21

10   9   8   7   6   5   4   3   2   1   First Printing

To Vijay, Ishani, and Sammy. All I have to do is
think of you and I remember that what I do have…
is extraordinary. Thank you for lighting the path.

—MK

To Sue, Mark, Reed, Vanessa, and Quinn. Happiness
is a kitchen full of family, doing the kitchen dance.

—PCK

Contents

Foreword

There has never been a time when guidance on how to effectively support children's mental health and well-being was needed as much as it is today.

Over the last ten years, we have seen a steady and significant increase in rates of depression and anxiety in young people compared to decades prior. In 2020, we experienced one of the most devastating global pandemics in modern history. The already growing problems with depression and anxiety in youth became exponentially worse.

The American Psychological Association recently published the report "Stress in America 2020: A National Mental Health Crisis." The survey included a sample of 1,026 teens ages 13–17, and it reports that Gen Z teens (ages 13–17) and Gen Z young adults (ages 18–23) are struggling with uncertainty, experiencing elevated stress, and reporting symptoms of depression. The pandemic brought to light our vulnerabilities—certainly economic, political, and social vulnerabilities, but also our individual vulnerabilities. We learned firsthand that with isolation and uncertainty, and few tools to buffer ourselves against them, both the mind and body suffer.

Perhaps this will be the impetus to change the trajectory of how we see and address the mental health crisis in youth. Perhaps now we will be more receptive to the idea that mental health is not something you are born either with or without; it must be built, nurtured, and supported every day, in all of us. And those of us who are more vulnerable will require early and targeted support.

Perhaps now we will be more likely to look to science to guide us in forging the path forward. The good news in all of this is that children can learn how to take charge of their emotions and be resilient rather than collapse with the weight of fear, loneliness, and uncertainty. The psychological interventions we have developed to facilitate this are effective and enduring, and there is a lower chance of relapse compared to medications.

One of these empirically supported interventions is the Coping Cat program for managing anxiety. With its FEAR plan and its behavioral experiments, Coping Cat is the most well-studied and effective behavioral intervention for anxiety in children and teens (Kendall and Hedtke 2006a, 2006b).

The Resilience Recipe, by Drs. Muniya Khanna and Philip Kendall, brings the components of Coping Cat to parents in a modern and science-informed approach. Why wait until a young adult develops difficulties with anxiety or depression? Why not provide a preventative basis to facilitate a child's healthy emotional development as a child? *The Resilience Recipe* does just that: it communicates, in a readable style, ways you can achieve realizable goals for your child. Each author is an expert and world-famous scholar on the topic of anxiety and mood difficulties in youth, and they combine their experiences and expertise to provide easy-to-implement and effective strategies for parents, including "conversation starters" that can help get you started in this resilience-building journey with your child. They also provide the principles behind the strategies, so you feel more informed about what to do and why. These principles are transdiagnostic—which means that they are effective in addressing a range of emotional difficulties, not just one target problem or a specific symptom (Barlow et al, 2017).

In this easy-to-read book, you will learn how to have the important conversations that can help your child build resilience against all types of emotional challenges and develop tools that will serve them for life. Every parent should be aware of the principles described in this manual.

—David H. Barlow PhD, ABPP

Emeritus Professor of Psychology and Psychiatry

Founder, Center for Anxiety and Related Disorders (CARD)

Boston University

Preface

We write this book with a sense of urgency. Our children are struggling, and it's our responsibility to do something about it. Currently, the lifetime prevalence rate of anxiety in children and adolescents in the US is a whopping 32 percent. Based on a recent epidemiological study, more than one in twenty children in the US have an anxiety disorder or depression. Eight out of ten are reporting excessive "stress" on a daily basis. From 2003 to 2011–2012, the rate of anxiety in children ages six to seventeen increased from 5.4 percent to 8.4 percent. According to the Centers for Disease Control and Prevention, the suicide rate among ten- to twenty-four-year-olds has *doubled* from 2007 to 2017, and suicide is now the second leading cause of death in fifteen- to twenty-year-olds. Since you've picked up this book, you probably know this and are concerned too. We applaud you for taking this active step, and we believe this book can give you the tools you need to give your child the gift of resilience. Not only the ability to respond well when faced with adversity, but also the ability to feel confident and capable *before* the challenges arise.

We are clinical psychologists and researchers who have dedicated our lives to understanding and treating anxiety and depression in children and teens. Our work is based on decades of clinical research with children and families across the country and around the world. There is much we still don't know, but we do know a lot about what helps and what does not. We also know that parents are in a great position to learn strategies and create a lifestyle that helps their children develop the skills to navigate stress and new challenges. Therapists, for an hour a week, can and do have a positive impact. School counselors and teachers, although often tasked with meeting the needs of large numbers of students and a wide range of tasks, are sources of great support. But the fact remains that during these years, parents have the greatest impact. Recent research has found that parents, by making changes to how they approach their children's stress and anxiety, help them as much as the children going to therapy (Lebowitz et al., 2020).

From our vantage point, from within research universities and specialty clinics, it has been frustrating to see that, despite the incredible need, current books, news outlets, and blog posts on parenting don't give parents a clear plan for what they can do at home. Mental health and its treatment are discussed in the media as abnormal and scary at worst, and at best, a mystery. We are always pleased to see characters on popular TV shows and films participating in talk therapy or medication management for mental health problems (famously in *The Sopranos, Monk, Glee, Silver Linings Playbook, Big Little Lies, Billions,* and *This Is Us,* among others), as this can be very powerful in normalizing and reducing stigma around seeking out mental health support. Still, those popular media representations often bestow on therapists or medications an almost magical power—something that can't be replicated in real life. The actor-portrayed, scripted therapist gives some key insight and asks one question that clears up everything. How does one find (or afford) a Dr. Wendy Rhoades? These dramas support and build on the popular mystique that surrounds mental health interventions and strategies. There are many "top ten" lists, "do's and don'ts," and personal stories published, but no formalized, clear guidance. Most frustrating are the articles and media that make recommendations and suggest strategies with no data to support that they are actually helpful long term. While parents today may be more open to seeking help for themselves and their children, they are no more likely to know what the help should look like or where to find it.

We take the blame. Having been stuck in the academic cycles of grant writing and publishing in research journals, we haven't done enough to inform and empower the general public. We thought our findings published in the *New England Journal of Medicine* and the *Journal of the American Medical Association* would make their way into the popular press. We hoped that in turn would lead to demand for new policies and systems for providing effective care and educating parents and caregivers. Unfortunately, that information was never broadcast to reach a wider audience.

What well-trained therapists offer isn't magical. They use well-understood and well-tested principles to guide their treatment—what we call *evidence-based treatment*. For over twenty years, therapists and counselors have used cognitive behavioral therapy (CBT) and the FEAR plan (more on that shortly) to help thousands of children and teens in clinics and schools around the world—but it's likely you haven't heard of these solutions. Until now. We have made it our mission to communicate to parents—and all adults working to support children and teens—everything we have learned through years of clinical work and research. We want to take the mystery out of stress and anxiety management so you can offer your children the gift of control over their emotions. In this book, we share with you the evidence-based, proven strategies for helping children build resilience. It is our hope that we will see strong foundations being built in homes across the country to manage stress and anxiety, helping our children lead lives full of passion, confidence, and well-being.

Why Are Our Kids More Stressed?

Although there are many possible causes for the increased rates of stress, anxiety, depression, and suicide, it's difficult to look backward in time to try to unravel them. Many studies have looked into the question, but the data are hard to interpret because most studies are retrospective and not well controlled. While we've gained a better understanding of risk factors and factors associated with anxiety and depression, which we'll discuss in later chapters, it's extremely difficult to find true causal links. Today's youth certainly face daunting new challenges. This post-9/11 generation was raised with the internet and smartphones; they have lived through a global financial crisis and one of the largest global pandemics in modern history. They have constant access to breaking news of natural disasters related to climate change, terrorism and mass shootings, racial and gender discrimination, economic uncertainty, and the pressures inherent in social media and a consumerist culture.

Then there is the ever-increasing pressure to achieve academic and athletic success. We have become all too familiar—almost desensitized—to the pressure-cooker analogy of our educational system. Experts predict that this situation will only worsen as the demand for college admissions and scholarships continues to grow in the next decade.

We know as parents that we are part of the problem. We allow our fears for our children's future to shape our parenting behaviors. So we find ourselves doubling down on perfectionism, setting extreme achievement expectations and demanding "peak" performance of our children from the time they are able to walk—letting our fears of failure and loss lead the way.

Instead of being more grateful, peaceful, and benevolent, instead of spreading knowledge, equality, and growth, we support (intentionally or unintentionally) more extreme in-groups and out-groups, widening socioeconomic, racial, and cultural inequities through exclusivity and competition, strengthening our commitment to establishing institutions of higher education as the gatekeepers for career opportunities and success, in hopes that our children will be among those who succeed.

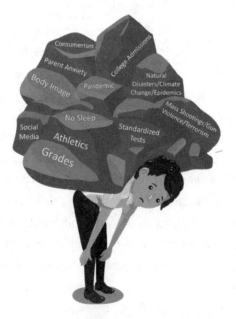

We parents are stressed by all of this too. And as parental stress rises, children's stress rises too, creating a compounding cycle of anxiety in the home. Truly, we are all living in an age of anxiety.

What Can We Do About It?

Looking forward, there are several very specific things that we can do better. A wide and impressive research literature describes how to help children and adolescents increase resilience; reduce intrusive, unwanted anxiety; and develop the skills to adapt to life's challenges without emotional unraveling. We can give our children this information and create opportunities to practice with them at home, with the right guidance. There are also strategies parents can learn to avoid the traps of a fear and failure mind-set that maintain anxiety themselves.

Dr. Kendall is the developer and author of the Coping Cat program, the most researched, well-established psychotherapy treatment program for anxiety in youth. His contribution to our understanding of childhood anxiety is immeasurable. Dr. Khanna is among the top clinical psychologists and researchers in anxiety and obsessive compulsive disorder (OCD) in children in the country and is a pioneer of web-based interventions and educational tools for children and parents with anxiety. We are honored and privileged to be able to say that we have been part of some of the most important research and writings in childhood anxiety over the last thirty years, establishing what is now the gold standard of care for children and teens with anxiety in mental health clinics, schools, and hospitals around the world.

The Coping Cat is based on the principles of CBT which has been rigorously studied in both children and adults and shown to be incredibly effective in helping manage mood and anxiety. We'll consider the principles of CBT and the key parts of effectively managing emotion in detail in the chapters that follow. The Coping Cat treatment program teaches kids the FEAR plan, using an acronym to help them remember four steps they can take to face fear, adversity, and self-doubt. (FEAR stands for What am I Feeling? Expecting bad things to happen? Attitudes and Actions that can help, and **R**esults and Rewards.) By walking themselves through the FEAR steps—which are based on the key components of CBT—children can reduce worry and anxiety and create a plan for approaching uncertainty rather than avoiding it.

In this book we will first explain the key principles for creating long-term resilience. Then we give guidance for applying the principles, walking you step by step through the FEAR plan. Our suggested conversation starters will help you start the conversations that communicate these principles in clear, kid-friendly language. Throughout, we share everything we have learned from our decades of research and clinical practice. We also want to acknowledge that we use the term "parent" throughout this book, but are speaking to all guardians, caregivers, and advocates in our children's lives.

Read on to learn the specific things you can do for your child, starting today.

—MK and PCK

PART 1

The Ingredients

CHAPTER 1

The Gift of Resilience

There is just no getting around that turning bad things into good things is totally up to you.

—Deepak Chopra

Our main goal in writing this book is to translate everything we know about resilience building and anxiety management in children from research and our clinical work into practical steps that you, as parents, can use at home. We feel it is important to give you not only a list of strategies, but the principles behind these strategies. Every strategy we suggest should have a rationale and guiding theory about how and why it helps. We know, from having trained thousands of therapists, that when you understand these principles you can feel more empowered to use the strategies to support your children than you would through trying to follow a series of "top ten tips." So before we get into detailing the FEAR plan and coping strategies to share with your child, we will first give you an overview of the principles of resilience. Times change, circumstances change, environments change, children mature, but the principles of human behavior stay the same. No matter your child's age or particular circumstances, you'll know what to do, because the principles will be the same.

Why Choose a CBT Approach?

The strategies for building resilience and coping with anxiety we describe in this book are based, again, on cognitive behavioral therapy (CBT). CBT has impressive research support and is a widely used intervention for many psychological problems. We recommend it for childhood (and adult) anxiety because it has been found to be incredibly effective. The Coping Cat—the most studied treatment for anxiety in children and teens—uses the acronym FEAR to guide children through safe, proven strategies to manage and decrease their stress and anxiety. It has also been found to reduce the risk of problems later in life, including depression, substance use, and anxiety disorders in adulthood. It is the gold-standard treatment—and best of all, anyone can learn and teach these strategies.

We want to avoid "preaching" CBT. The practices of mindfulness, acceptance and commitment therapy, dialectical behavioral therapy, Buddhist philosophy, and other world philosophies share many of the same principles. This underscores the truth that specific terminology is less important than the universal principles that underlie them. We are using science to guide which strategies and recommendations we make, and CBT provides a blueprint that is easy to understand and has proven effective in helping children build resilience.

The goal of CBT, as with most psychological theories of well-being, is to help people become aware of their thoughts and patterns of behavior that may be maintaining negative emotions and low self-worth. Awareness of our patterns takes away the strength and automatic nature of our response. It gives us time to consider and choose alternative ways of thinking and behaviors that allow a different, more adaptive, positive response, so we can create a lifetime of peace and joy.

The cognitive behavioral theory on which CBT is based has a rich scientific and theoretical history that has survived the ages. Understanding the principles of this theory will give you a strong foundation on which to build resilience at home.

The Foundation: Cognitive Behavioral Theory

Cognitive behavioral theory is the foundation for the strategies and recommendations we discuss in this book. This theory combines the key principles of behaviorism, or learning theory, that evolved through the work of such great scholars as Skinner, Pavlov, Watson, Thorndike, and Bandura, together with cognitive theory, as penned by Aaron T. Beck and expanded by others including Ellis and Meichenbaum. As with any theory of human personality, cognitive behavioral theory must address the hows and whys of human behavior and emotion. Why do we feel what we feel? Why do we do what we do? Let's break down this model and dig in a little further. We'll see how our thoughts, learning history, and biology work together to influence our emotions and our actions, and subsequently shape our understanding of ourselves and our world. Then we'll discuss how we can apply these principles to equip and empower our children to be resilient in the face of any challenge.

Our Thoughts (Cognition)

Why do we feel what we feel? Cognitive theory suggests that our thoughts (cognition) have a very powerful influence on our behavioral, emotional, and physical response. It recognizes that our thoughts about ourselves and our situations, or our interpretation of our situation, can change our experience of that situation. We do not all have the same response to the same situation, because for each of us our thoughts, or how we interpret the situation, are different.

Cognitive theory brings to light an incredibly powerful and key element for understanding human well-being. It highlights that *it is our thoughts that create our emotional experience, our "reality"—not our situation or the outside world.* Though we may have unimaginable wealth, if we're focused on a loss, we can feel hopeless and deprived. We can be surrounded by friends and family, but if focused on a rejection, we can feel alone and unloved. This reminds us that there are really no "truths," outside of the laws of nature and science, that are "real," or fact. Our laws, values, priorities, beliefs—we have either chosen them, agreed to them, or accepted them. This implies that we can challenge anything that we are thinking.

For example: I value the opinion of my boss, and I feel anxiety when I anticipate negative feedback. What are my rules of "failure" and "success"? Where did these rules come from? Do I really agree with them? Are there alternate ways to define or measure failure and success? What do I define as negative feedback? Where did these definitions and rules come from? Is there another perspective or an alternate way to think about this feedback?

Many of us live our lives in reaction mode—simply going from situation to gut reaction. This assumes that we have no control over our inner experience—that the world is acting on us and we are just trying to react in whatever way we can to survive.

Situation → Emotion

Sitting in class → Anxious

But from the perspective of cognitive theory, we see that it is actually our thoughts that are creating our emotional experience. The world is happening around us, we are interpreting it, and that interpretation is bringing about our emotional experience.

Situation → Thoughts → Emotion

Sitting in class → *If I make a mistake, everyone will think I'm stupid.* → Anxious

This is our greatest weakness—our kryptonite. Because we have the ability to create an emotional response just with our thoughts, we can create negative emotions without leaving our chair! Unlike other mammals on the planet (as far as we know), we don't need a negative situation or experience to create a negative emotional response. We don't need to actually be chased by a bear—we can just anticipate this happening, or reflect on a prior negative experience, or imagine one. We can feel anxious and miserable, anytime and anywhere, regardless of what is going on around us.

Situation → Thoughts → Emotion

Sunday night at home → *If I make a mistake, everyone will think I'm stupid.* → Anxious

But *this is also our superpower.* Because we can reflect, anticipate, and choose the focus of our thoughts, we have the power to choose our emotional response as well as our behavioral response. *We are able to choose our response.* Therefore, we determine the distance between the emotion we *want* and the emotion we *have.* We can create the emotional response we want, as soon as we choose the interpretation that supports it.

Situation → Chosen Thoughts → Emotion

Sunday night at home → *Ugh, school tomorrow. It's okay; if I make a mistake, it will feel bad but then the feeling will pass; I'm just learning.* → Content

Our Learning History

Why do we do what we do? Behavioral theory suggests that our behaviors, or our actions, are a result of what we learned from the consequences of past and ongoing experiences, or our *learning history.* For example, if you told a lie and it got you out of trouble, from that experience you learned that lying is a behavior that can be effective in getting you out of trouble. Once learned, the behavior repeats in the face of similar stimuli or circumstances. You might choose lying whenever there's a chance, and with repetition you learn that it is a helpful strategy. Over time, the relationship between the behavior and circumstance strengthens, and eventually we form patterns of behavior, sometimes called habits. You may become fluent in lying in more and more types of situations. Learning theory explains how our habits come to be, and why, despite what we know to be the most logical or "right" thing to do, our behaviors follow old patterns, and these can be so difficult to change.

Key to learning theory is the notion of shaping; that every response is *shaped* by the consequences of that response. For instance, if someone says "You look great in blue," you may find yourself wearing more blue. If you felt good when lots of people "liked" your photo on social media, you may be quicker to post another similar photo. Your behavior was shaped, in this case increased (behavioral science would say it was *reinforced*), by the positive feedback you received. If you feel relaxed and less troubled by work when you watch TV, you may be quicker to turn on the TV. Bottom line: If what you do makes you feel good or feel less distressed, you are more likely to do it again—even if the behavior is negative.

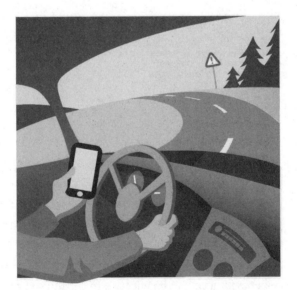

We often find ourselves checking our phones, even when we know it's not the right time. Phones offer a lot of positive reinforcement for checking—we feel reassured that we are "liked" and included, and/or that we are not missing out on important information. Checking our phone also offers a brief escape from difficult tasks.

And yes, the opposite is true—if what you do makes you feel uncomfortable or distressed, you'll be less likely to do it again. If someone makes a rude or jokingly negative comment about your shoes, you may find yourself less inclined to wear those shoes again. If you get a critical and harsh evaluation for an essay you wrote, you'll be less likely to want to start writing another essay.

This process gets more complex. If the consequence or outcome of your response is that something bad *stops* happening, you will also be more likely to do it again. For example, if you find that when you get up early, your dog doesn't have accidents on the carpet, you may become more likely to get up early. The reduction of something negative is also reinforcing! We call this *negative reinforcement*—you increasingly respond in this way not because something *positive* is happening, but because something negative is *not* happening. Thus we could predict that if a parent *stops* criticizing their child when the child is in their room, the child may be more likely to stay in their room.

This also explains why each of us behaves differently even in the same circumstances. We do not all respond the same way to the same situations because our past consequences, or what we have learned, are different.

Our Neurobiology

The cognitive and behavioral theories are then integrated with a third theory: the neurobiological theory of emotion. We have learned a lot about the molecular, cellular, genetic, and anatomic correlates of emotion, and we continue to learn more. For example, we know that our brains are prewired to scan, prepare, and act when in danger through the well-known fight-or-flight response—a neurobiological response intended to protect us from danger and then bring our bodies back to baseline.

We also have learned that genetic vulnerabilities or predispositions underlie not only our physical characteristics, like hair color and height, but also our emotional characteristics, like vulnerability to anxiety and/

or depression. This means those with predispositions to anxiety or depression are more vulnerable to experiencing anxiety or depressed mood than those without such predispositions. They may have a more frequent or more intense physiological response to threats both real and imagined, becoming anxious and avoidant or too often falling into hopelessness and withdrawal or a "hibernation" response. Children vulnerable to anxiety may have heightened sensitivity and have more frequent or more intense fight-or-flight responses than those without this vulnerability.

The three theories combine to form a comprehensive model in which each of these influences the others. Cognitive behavioral theory purports that we are who we are, and feel what we feel, and do what we do, because of the interplay of our thoughts, learning history, and biology. Put another way, our thoughts interpret our past and present and influence our behavioral and physiological responses, which create our emotions, and vice versa, and in every direction!

Over time, we develop enduring patterns of interpretation of events (our stories) and enduring patterns of reacting physiologically and emotionally (feelings) that produce patterns of behavior (actions) that can be either adaptive (working well for us) or maladaptive (not working well for us).

Cognitive Behavioral Theory of Emotion

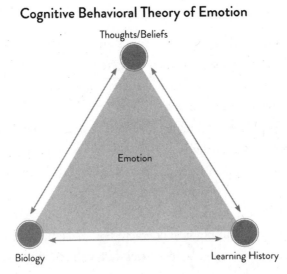

Notice, in this model, that the situation or circumstance is not the primary driver of the experience. We can see how our beliefs and our habits influence us in every moment and potentially create more of the same experience, regardless of the situation.

Beliefs + Biological Predispositions + Past Learning →

I'm not smart enough + Fight/Flight/Freeze + Felt embarrassed after making a mistake →

Our response is more dependent on our preexisting beliefs, biology, and learning history than on the situation itself. Our outcome, or our experience, depends as much on our approach to the situation as on the situation itself.

Cumulatively, these experiences make up what we look back on and think of as our life. They make up the stories that become the foundation of our identity. If we choose negative stories, we will find ourselves in more emotional distress more often and subsequently choosing negative behaviors, like withdrawal or aggression, that lead to more negative outcomes, further maintaining our negative interpretations and lower self-esteem, and on and on.

Now the good news. This also means that regardless of our situation, we still are in the driver's seat of our thoughts, behaviors, and emotions. We don't have to just react to situations; we can choose our response. We can choose to face any situation without becoming overwhelmed. *We can keep things in perspective, adapt, bounce back—be resilient.* Even better, we can create the experiences we want, rather than waiting for circumstances to create our experience. Cumulatively creating the life we choose, rather than simply succumbing to life as it presents itself.

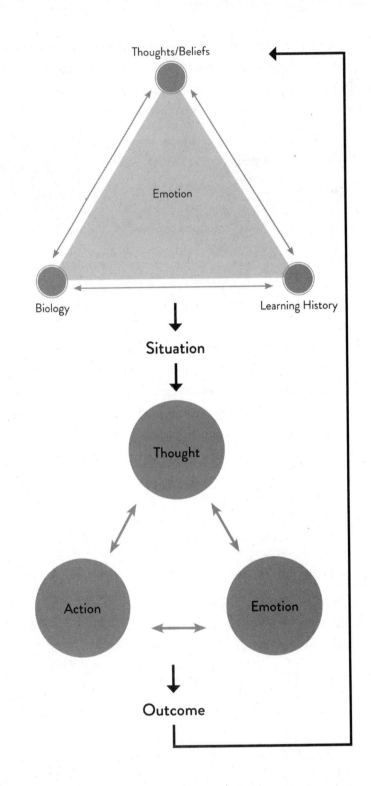

Beliefs + Biological Predispositions + Past Learning → Situation→ Thoughts → Emotion

Learning something new involves making mistakes + Fight/Flight/ Freeze + It is uncomfortable but it's okay, everyone makes mistakes → Sunday night at home → *If I make a mistake, it will feel bad but then the feeling will pass; I'm just learning.* → Calm

Can Resilience Be Taught to Children? If So, How?

Resilience can and should be taught to children. There are simple changes in how your child approaches new, uncomfortable, or challenging situations that can absolutely lessen how stressed or down they feel. If you can share this understanding with your child, you will be giving them an invaluable gift. The gift of awareness and agency over their emotions. The gift of resilience. In fact, the earlier you share this with them, the easier it will be for them to develop habits that feed confidence, allowing them to live empowered.

The Principles of Resilience

Resilience is being equipped to approach life with confidence and the ability to respond adaptively in times of adversity. Developing an awareness of and compassion for our emotional and physiological experience, cultivating a mind-set of growth and flexibility, practicing prosocial behaviors and positive ways to problem solve and approach challenges— these are the ingredients of resilience, and the FEAR plan is the recipe. In this book we will walk you step by step through these key ingredients, and you'll use the FEAR acronym to teach your children these same principles in a way that's easy to understand and remember.

Developing Awareness and Compassion

The first and most important step is to help your child understand the connection between their mind, body, feelings, and behaviors; to help them become aware of their own patterns—the way their body responds to different emotions, which thoughts pop up in different situations, and which behaviors have become habits—and to observe these without judgment. Awareness will give them enough distance from the situation to be able to think about how they would like to respond. Compassion about one's emotional and physiological experience takes away the surrounding fear and guilt, creating enough of an opening to try something different.

Cultivating a Mind-set of Growth and Flexibility

The next goal will be to help them see how their thoughts and behaviors are influencing how they feel and what they experience in their world. Having a mind-set that there is no failure, or rejection—just opportunities to grow and learn—will equip them to be able to bounce back when they face a tough test, or a betrayal from a friend, or any negative event. Over time it will become more automatic for them to view challenges as a problem to be solved, and they'll become flexible enough to adapt and turn challenges into opportunities to learn and grow. They'll know that they can choose their focus—*what do I have, what can I do?* rather than *what have I lost?*

Adopting a Lifestyle of Approach

This is perhaps the most crucial, yet most often skipped, ingredient. Doing the thing that has been avoided, or purposefully planning to approach challenges, is a key step in rewiring our brains, creating new connections, and weakening old ones. Unless your child practices the "new" or "chosen" behavior, their brain won't really "learn" anything new. For example, they can change how they've been thinking about a situation (*It's okay if I make a mistake; everyone makes mistakes*) but if they don't change the behavior that has been maintaining the worry (say, they're still not raising their hand in class), they'll still experience the same fight-or-flight response and can fall back into the cycle of worry about failure and humiliation every time they are faced with a similar situation.

This step is so often skipped for three main reasons:

- It is impossible to "make" someone do something they don't want to do, and it's difficult for people to "choose" to do something they've been actively avoiding.

- It's difficult to create opportunities for practicing preplanned challenges.

- Parents often have been working so hard to minimize anxiety or stressful events that it becomes difficult and distressing to reverse course and start pushing their child to do the things that could spark anxiety.

In later chapters we will discuss how to overcome these obstacles. For now, keep this principle in mind: *approach* is almost always better than *avoidance*. Whenever possible, encouraging your child to approach challenges, even if they might fail or feel disappointed, will help them become more resilient long term.

If you create a lifestyle of approach, your child will experience less anxiety and more resilience in all types of situations. We use the term *lifestyle* because it may seem, when we recommend strategies, that the goal is to target only specific fears with practice. It is true that targeting fears that are long-standing and frequent are worth targeting and the FEAR plan practices will help. But we hope that parents will encourage approach for all types of everyday situations:

"Should we try it?"	"Yes."
"Should I call?"	"Yes."
"Do you think it will work?"	"I don't know, but let's try."
"What if no one is there?"	"Well, we'll see and make the best of it either way."

	"Our chances are good."
"It's too late."	"Maybe, but we'll be glad we at least tried."
"It's going to be so hard."	"It might be hard, but it won't be anything you can't handle."

A lifestyle of approach builds up a reservoir of experience at tackling challenges, making new ones increasingly less daunting.

The Ultimate Gift: Security

Our job as parents is relatively straightforward, although not easy. It's our job to support, guide, appreciate, and encourage. By following the principles described in these chapters, you'll be guiding and supporting your child in ways that will help them thrive. This is the greatest gift we can give to another, and it's one a parent can offer better than anyone else. The gift of security. Not in terms of safety from harm—sadly, you won't be able to prevent or protect them from all harm—but security in knowing you are there to support them. The gift of knowing you'll always be there to help, comfort, trust, appreciate, and understand them unconditionally, exactly as they are.

The absence of any of these things (support, guidance, encouragement, security) can have long-term impact. Resilience requires confidence in our ability to recover from adversity. Remember from learning theory that the environment and the consequences of our experiences are constantly shaping our view of ourselves and our world. If your child has *learned* over time that they are vulnerable or incompetent, that they lack skill and judgment, it will be impossible for them to form a mind-set of confidence and competence. Your child cannot feel confident if they have not often experienced appreciation and competence. Appreciate and encourage them when they approach a task, even if they fail. Becoming quickly frustrated, upset, or yelling, or moving in too quickly to remove the obstacle, sends a message that they should be ashamed or afraid of failure. It's extremely difficult to feel self-confident and fear failure at the same time.

In your efforts to teach, communicate, and practice these principles with your child, your results will vary. It's best not to measure your child's or your own "success." Rather, in line with our principles, just know that there is no real benchmark for success. You'll know you're doing a good job communicating these principles to your child simply because you genuinely intend to do and give as much as you can. And you'll know your child is doing a good job in learning these skills because all children naturally learn and grow from what they hear, see, and do. You cannot expect to change anyone. We don't have access to changing anyone outside of ourselves. Certainly, you have influence, as we've acknowledged. But our children are not ours to mold. We are not *making* them more resilient; rather, we are giving them what we can to allow resilience to develop.

In the chapters ahead, we will provide an overview of the FEAR plan and show you how you can communicate these principles to your child by using this simple acronym.

Key Takeaways

In every situation, how we respond is influenced by three things:

- Our thoughts: Our beliefs about ourselves and our interpretation of the experience. It is our thoughts that create our reality, not our situation or the outside world.

- Our biology: Our evolutionarily-shaped physiology and genetic predispositions.

- Our learned behaviors: What we have learned from past experiences and those behaviors that have become habits.

Being aware and in control of our response enables us to take charge of our journey—to create what we want to experience rather than just reacting as things unfold.

Resilience is being equipped to approach life with confidence and the ability to respond adaptively in times of adversity.

Resilience develops when these three things are in place:

- An awareness of and compassion for one's emotional and physiological experience

- A mind-set of growth and flexibility

- A lifestyle of approach

These three key ingredients of resilience are communicated through a memorable acronym—FEAR—that helps kids use them. The next chapters walk you through teaching your child the FEAR plan.

CHAPTER 2

Understanding Anxiety

Never say never, because limits, just like fear, are often an illusion.

—Michael Jordan

Think of the best slice of pizza you've ever had. What it smelled like, how it tasted when you bit into it. The gooey, warm cheese; the sweet, tangy tomato sauce. Any chance you are salivating right now? Your body, in thinking about the pizza, started the digestion process—even though you're not sitting in front of any actual pizza. Similarly, just by thinking about an uncomfortable or scary moment, your body can start a fight-or-flight process without needing to actually be in a dangerous situation.

Unlike any other animal (as far as we have conclusively determined), humans can imagine, anticipate, and reflect on danger, producing the physiological fight-or-flight response without being faced with an immediate threat. Just a thought can trigger a cascade of physiological events involving the sympathetic nervous system—heart starts racing, cortisol levels rise, palms begin to sweat, and muscles tense. What we call "anxiety" is our interpretation of the arousal we feel in our body that comes when the fight-or-flight response begins.

Our human ability to reflect, plan, and anticipate is both our greatest strength and our greatest weakness. It allows us to learn from past mistakes and improve future outcomes. Our ability to create and imagine in our minds allows novel ideas and innovation. But our complex and imaginative minds also allow us to linger longer on disappointments, interpret neutral experiences as negative ones, and initiate fight-or-flight responses from mere stories. This can be particularly damaging in today's world, in which we are bombarded by stories and reminders of threats in many forms. We can be in a state of heightened arousal, or experiencing "anxiety," all day long, even though we are not in immediate danger.

Think of what happens for most animals. As soon as a deer realizes that a predator may be approaching, its fight-or-flight response is triggered. Now, in full hormonal surge, the deer runs as fast as it ever has to safety. Once in a safe spot, the deer's body calms down and returns to a baseline state. In the moments that follow, the deer is not reflecting on its experience, not planning its next escape route, not ruminating about its inability to avoid the danger in the first place. Certainly this has drawbacks. The deer's inability to reflect and plan leaves it as vulnerable to future attacks as before. But we can also see the benefits. The deer is not in a heightened state of arousal throughout the day. Its body spends more time at baseline than not.

How do we gain control over our minds and bodies so that we don't overdo anticipating danger or continually initiate our fight-or-flight response? As we mentioned in chapter 1, the first step is by building awareness.

The Worry Cycle

Understanding anxiety—what it is, where it comes from, what maintains it, and what weakens it—will put you and your child in a position to know what to do next instead of just feeling overwhelmed and reacting instinctively. Even better, you'll understand how to create a lifestyle that can reset the system, change its course, and make anxiety less and less of a threat.

When it comes to fear or anxiety, a predictable cycle emerges. We're going to call it the *worry cycle*. When we anticipate a threat—even if it is just potential discomfort, not danger (for example, *They'll think I'm stupid*)—a "what if" thought pops up and our fight-or-flight system kicks in (increased arousal, heart rate, sweating, muscle tension). We are prewired to find a way to either prevent harm or protect from future

The Worry Cycle

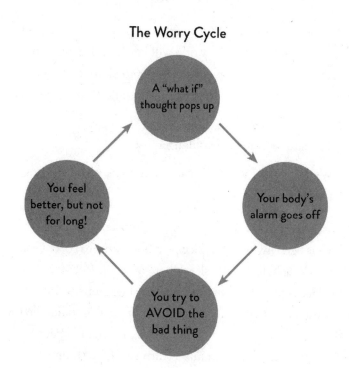

harm—our instinct tells us to flee (*I'll start working on this tomorrow*). What we call *worry* is our brain scanning for danger and searching for ideas about how we could defend ourselves from what might be out there. If and when we do retreat, we gain quick relief, and our body's alarm system turns off and goes back to baseline.

This perceived "relief" is incredibly reinforcing, as learning theory would have predicted—through negative reinforcement. With repetition, our body learns that relief comes from retreat or avoidance. We tend to detect and interpret danger (or discomfort) and to seek relief through escape, thus reinforcing a cycle of anxiety and avoidance. More and more situations start to feel dangerous.

Left unimpeded, the fight-or-flight response cycle can become overactive and interfering. Our brain becomes focused on all the bad things that are happening and starts to expect bad things to happen again. After a while, we begin planning ways to "fix" it, prevent it from happening, or avoid it completely (*Maybe I'll skip school today*) before anything has happened.

Thinking back to cognitive behavioral theory, this means that our beliefs about ourselves and the world will be changing over time as well. Unfortunately, the cycle of avoidance leads to changes in one's self-efficacy (confidence in one's own ability to handle things), because each time we avoid, we reinforce two beliefs:

1. The situation really was dangerous!

2. We are vulnerable—we can't handle new, difficult, or uncomfortable situations.

Let's see the worry cycle in action. We'll take an example of a young teen who has been invited to a sleepover. She wants to go, but she worries that she won't be able to fall asleep there and will feel scared and alone all night. Her internal alarm goes off. So she listens to her alarm and interprets that she is vulnerable and may not be able to handle the situation. She decides not to go. She feels better in that moment because of her decision, but her body and mind learn two false things:

1. Sleepovers are dangerous. Bad stuff can happen at sleepovers, like not being able to fall asleep, missing your mom and dad, or being scared in someone else's house.

2. She is vulnerable. Unlike others, she can't handle sleepovers.

Next time she gets invited to a sleepover, her alarm will go off, and she'll worry. If she again interprets danger and decides not to go, she will reinforce the cycle and make the next sleepover that much more difficult. She won't have had the experience of learning that the situation wasn't dangerous—that it just caused her to feel uncomfortable because it was new and there was uncertainty. She'll also not have gained the experience (learning) that she can handle new, difficult, and uncomfortable situations.

Over time, her brain may start to scan for "danger" about nighttime in general. The thought *What if I can't fall asleep?* may start popping up more often.

We are quick to assume that it's the situation (a book report is due in school, there's a big game coming up) that makes us worry. But

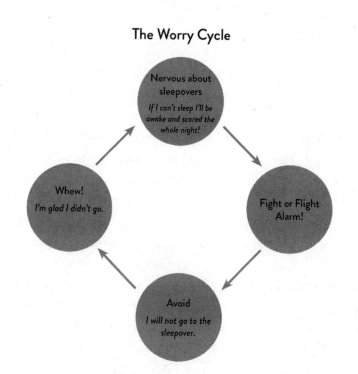

The Worry Cycle

Nervous about sleepovers
If I can't sleep I'll be awake and scared the whole night!

Fight or Flight Alarm!

Avoid
I will not go to the sleepover.

Whew!
I'm glad I didn't go.

actually it's our thoughts about the situation that cause our bodies to go into protection mode. We want things to go smoothly, so as soon as we think *What if it doesn't?*, our body's alarm goes off and we go straight into planning our escape. We try to make sure the bad things don't happen, but that's exactly why the worry keeps coming back—we're teaching our brain that these things (like messing up) are dangerous. However, they're *not* dangerous; rather, they are uncomfortable, and we can survive discomfort.

After a while, our bodies learn, incorrectly, that we *can't handle* discomfort and that we *are* in danger. Ironically, all the planning, prevention, and avoidance of bad things serves only to increase stress and anxiety. If we continue to avoid situations, the cycle of anxiety continues, and the anxious thoughts are reinforced. With more anxious thoughts and physiological symptoms and more avoidance, soon there's more interference with everyday activities. At its worst, this cycle stops us from having fun, experiencing freedom, and enjoying important and meaningful life experiences.

We want to highlight that avoidance can take many forms beyond just skipping out on new situations that make us anxious. Avoidance can take the form of over-planning, over-preparing, checking, seeking reassurance, procrastinating, distracting, even trying not to think about something—all of these offer temporary relief but are ineffective in relieving stress and anxiety. Even worse, these avoidance strategies create new problems. In addition to reinforcing our anxiety, they have their own negative consequences. Putting off tasks too long, asking too many (or too few) questions, spending too many hours looking for the "right" answer, or too many nights "trying not to think about it," can leave kids with lost friendships, lower grades, missed opportunities, and lost sleep—all of which create new challenges and new worries.

Here's a little experiment: Think of a pink giraffe. Now make the giraffe smile and dance. Now stop thinking about the giraffe. Try not to think about it. Think about anything *but* the pink giraffe. Whatever you do, don't think about a pink giraffe. You can see that it's impossible to not think about something when the thing is in the sentence. The sentence *Try not to think about* X flies through your mind as you are instructing yourself, so it will be part of the thought. If you check—*Is it still there?*—it will be. If you start thinking of a plan to make it go away, then it will be there the whole time and can cause even more anxiety because it's not going away, despite your plan. If you try to distract yourself with an activity, it will interrupt your activity. The only way to really stop thinking about the pink giraffe is by letting it pop up and accepting that it is there, without judgment. Your mind attended to it, but it's not important, so you don't need to put energy into trying to make it go away. No additional instructions relating to it in your self-talk. Then go back to focusing on what you were doing. *What was I doing before the thought popped up?* Every time your mind wanders back to the giraffe, let it be there, and quickly move to what you were doing before that thought popped up. Over time, your mind won't be actively engaged with it and it will fade away. This concept of accepting anxious thoughts, without judgment, letting them come and go, not avoiding or trying to push them away, is among the key elements of mindfulness-based stress reduction and acceptance and commitment therapies; it's also consistent with our cognitive behavioral perspective.

There is one other interesting and important fact about anxiety: once our brain has felt the relief it gets from avoidance, it seems to almost hunger for that relief. In therapy we sometimes give this a name, like "the hungry puppy" or "the bully," because, like a hungry puppy, our brain figures out how to get what it wants from you and keeps coming back for more. Keep giving the puppy what it wants—because it's begging and insistently persistent—and soon you'll have a voracious dog that won't leave you alone. It's as though your brain has figured out what it can remind you of to get your attention—and feed its need for relief.

For example, if someone gets particularly anxious in social situations, their brain will seem to pay more attention to these situations in general. They may think often about negative outcomes in social situations (*They won't like me; I'll be sitting by myself the whole time*). The more they attempt to avoid such situations or relieve the worry, the more they notice feeling uncomfortable every time they face or anticipate a social situation. Over time, they may build up different ways to avoid. For example, they may develop a need to over-prepare for presentations, become quick to look away or avoid eye contact, not volunteer for tasks that would put them in the spotlight, or create routines that don't involve other people.

Awareness of your own avoidance pattern can be very useful. In the example, when a social engagement is coming up, the person can be alert that anxiety is sure to come up. They'll know what it will feel like, and what will probably happen next. They can let the thoughts come and go, without judgment, and feel less upset or frustrated when they come because they knew they were coming. They can even decide to do something differently next time. In our FEAR plan chapters, we will help you help your child get fluent at identifying their patterns, their most common "what ifs," and their most common avoidance behaviors. Identifying these will give them the time and perspective to challenge them; only then can they create change. In other words, by knowing their cycle, they can break the cycle.

Is Anxiety in Kids Different?

Regardless of age, fight or flight works on the same principles. We are all hard-wired to not like uncertainty. Most of the time our fight-or-flight system works beautifully. Our built-in alarm system makes us jump back quickly when we step off a curb and suddenly see a car speeding toward us. We don't have to think *There's a car coming! I should jump back!*—we just jump. We are designed to scan for and protect ourselves from threat. This is true for both children (after a certain age) and adults, and this serves us well from an evolutionary perspective. If we just went up to a snake and picked it up, that could be dangerous! Experiencing some anticipation of threat also helps us to prepare for important things. If we didn't think about outcomes, we might not organize our day, study for tests, or prepare for important events, and we wouldn't do as well. Our fight-or-flight response speeds up heart rate, breathing, muscle readiness, glandular function, and circulation of the blood. In short, it gets the body ready to protect itself when danger is identified—and this is good. But a lot of times it gets it *wrong*. It becomes a problem when the alarm goes off when there is no real danger, or when it goes off too often—when it's a false alarm.

When your child experiences anxiety, they are anticipating or attending to perceived threat—a common human reaction. There is nothing weird or wrong with the particular nature of the danger being anticipated or the specific kinds of worries your child has. They may sound extreme or even silly, but the content of the fear is typically universal. We are all concerned about many of the same things, and most of them have an evolutionary basis.

The focus of our fears, however, does change with development. Babies are less developed cognitively, so their fight-or-flight response is working on primal instincts, instinctively reacting to unfamiliar faces or loud noises. In toddlers, there is normal separation anxiety when separated from their trusted caregiver. This can take the form of fussiness, agitation, not eating, or crying. Young children may fear imaginary threats, like a monster under the bed. Once they are old enough to think in the abstract, they worry about things they have heard about but never experienced, like kidnappers, natural disasters, or death. Older children and teens have started developing meaningful social relationships outside of immediate family, which brings on new worries about friendships and rejection.

Your child may worry mostly about their friendships, or mostly about grades and performance, or maybe they worry all the time about everything. "What if I get in trouble?" "What if I fail?" "What if I'm late?" "What if I forget?" "What if they laugh?" There isn't a problem with the logic behind how they see the world. It's not that they don't know that it's really unlikely that they will get kidnapped in the middle of the night. The trouble is, their body, when attending to that thought, is giving them an alarm signal—a signal that is extreme, and difficult for them to ignore, and hinders them from noticing that they are not in danger, that the thing they are anticipating is either not dangerous or very unlikely to happen. Watching a show, playing on their computer or phone, taking a nap, or skipping school might be what they choose to do to feel better in the short term, but they might be increasing the likelihood that they'll experience even more anxiety the next time they are faced with a similar challenge.

Normal Anxiety versus Excessive Anxiety

Parents often ask us how to tell the difference between normal fears and excessive anxiety. Children who struggle with anxiety are vulnerable to experiencing frequent fight-or-flight "alarms" and/or have developed a cycle that creates a near-constant need for predictability, perfection, and avoiding "discomfort." Their thinking becomes hyperfocused on all the bad things that are happening or could happen in a situation, and they begin planning ways to try to "fix" it, prevent it from happening, or avoid it completely. After a while, their body and mind learn, incorrectly, that they can't handle discomfort and that they actually *are* in danger. All the planning, prevention, and avoidance of bad things, ironically, serves only to increase stress and anxiety.

How can you tell if your child's anxiety is normal or excessive—or even, perhaps, indicative of an anxiety disorder? A basic guideline is to think of three factors: intensity, frequency, and interference.

How *intense* is the anxiety or stress your child is experiencing? Does it seem more intense than what you might expect for someone that age in the same situation? Or is it in the range of what you might expect, but given that there are stressful things going on lately, they've just been more anxious than usual?

Is anxiety too *frequent*? That is, has it become an issue more often than you'd like—almost every day, more days than not? Does the anxiety come up almost every time your child is faced with the situation or thing that disturbs them?

Is the anxiety getting in the way of your child's day to day activities? When thinking of *interference*, think of how anxiety might be getting in the way of life. At school, how well is your child doing academically, athletically, or socially? Is their anxiety having an impact on any of these? How much do they enjoy going to school? How much are they getting out of the experience?

You can think also about your child's relationships with peers: is it difficult for your child to make new friends, keep friends, or enjoy time with friends because of anxiety? What about family relationships? Is anxiety making things tense at home, where family members are getting into arguments or feeling like they have to "work around" the child's anxiety?

How much is anxiety bothering your child themself? Do they seem very distressed because the anxiety is intense? Does your child notice how difficult things are in different situations? Is it hard for your child to stop feeling anxious or to distract themself from their anxiety once it starts?

It's not always easy to distinguish between normal anxiety and an anxiety disorder, so here's an example of the difference: Consider a child who feels nervous about an upcoming school test. This motivates him to study for the test. Although he still feels some anxiety during the test, he is able to concentrate and complete the test. And after the test is over, he does not continue worrying about how well he did, and he can rest and enjoy his activities. In contrast, a child with an anxiety disorder may experience high levels of anxiety prior to the test. Fear of failure may lead him to try to avoid the test altogether. During the test, he has a hard time concentrating and completing the test; his worries and fears are just too persistent and intense. After the test, he remains upset and unable to move on to other activities, because he can't stop thinking about how he did.

Anxiety is considered excessive and possibly an anxiety disorder if it is:

- Persistent—lasting for months
- Uncontrollable—coming up in a variety of situations throughout the day on most days
- Linked to avoidance that interferes with daily living
- Intense and distressing—more intense than for most kids of that age

If your child's anxiety is coming up only once in a while, and you aren't convinced that it's much more than normal or getting in the way just yet, please keep reading. Everyday stress can be difficult for a child to manage, and how you handle it can influence how they feel and how they learn to handle stress as they grow. This book can help you manage your child's anxiety and can also help when it may qualify as an anxiety disorder.

Anxiety Disorders

Anxiety disorders are the most common mental health conditions in adults and children, with between 10 and 15 percent of kids struggling with excessive anxiety. To put this into perspective, if your child goes to a school where there are thirty students in each grade, it's likely that three or four of the kids in each grade will have excessive anxiety. And if the entire school has five hundred students, of these five hundred, there could be seventy-five or more children with excessive anxiety. These numbers are concerning, but there is good news: there are effective strategies for helping kids manage their anxiety and change its course. We will describe these strategies in this book, step by step, to help you communicate and practice them with your child.

Kids who struggle with excessive anxiety generally find anxiety-related interference impacting many areas of their lives. They may experience low self-esteem, social isolation, limited social skills, problems with school work, excess stress about performance, and difficulty launching into adulthood. Unlike behavior problems (acting out, hyperactivity) and even, to some degree, depression, anxiety is often overlooked, partly because it is experienced by everyone to some degree so it's considered somewhat normal. There can also be long-term physical and emotional problems; though the connection often goes unrecognized, the physical ailments that may stem from anxiety disorder include hypertension, sleep disturbance and resulting fatigue, gastrointestinal problems, respiratory illness, arthritis, skin problems—the list goes on.

Over the long term, anxiety is associated with higher risk of depression, substance use problems, and other anxiety disorders in adulthood.

Our Symptom Checker is available on our website at http://www.CopingCatParents.com or for download at http://www.newharbinger.com/46967. You'll find descriptions and brief checklists to identify different categories of anxiety. We also offer a parent-training program on our website, http://www.CopingCatParents.com. The strategies we describe in this book will be helpful for any and all of these types of anxiety, because all anxiety works in kind of the same way, so we fight it the same way no matter what the content. The Symptom Checker may be a good place to start if you are trying to decide whether to seek support from a professional in addition to your developing a solid understanding of anxiety and the strategies in this book.

The information in this book and websites is not intended nor implied to constitute medical advice, diagnosis, or a substitute for this advice or treatment. To really establish whether or not your child has a diagnosable anxiety disorder, you should visit or speak to a qualified health service provider.

Key Takeaways

Our brains are designed to protect us from harm. What we call anxiety is our interpretation of the arousal we feel in our body that comes with the fight-or-flight response.

Just because we feel this arousal doesn't mean we are in danger. It's more often a false alarm. If we respond with avoidance in response to a false alarm, we may be inadvertently reinforcing more false alarms. And if we prevent or avoid negative outcomes or emotions too often, our brain learns two wrong things:

- New, difficult, or uncomfortable situations are dangerous.

- We can't handle new, difficult, or uncomfortable situations.

When you put off action or even if you get stuck planning and not doing, that can keep you in a worry cycle. Your mind is reading from your inaction that you are not okay—you need relief—so your body starts feeling more anxious, making it even harder to get going.

If you are concerned and wanting to assess the severity of problem anxiety, think about the intensity, frequency, and interference of your stress and anxiety. We suggest speaking with a healthcare professional who can help make an assessment and offer recommendations for next steps.

CHAPTER 3

The FEAR Plan:
Steps to Breaking the Cycle

Courage is resistance to fear, mastery of fear, not absence of fear.

—Mark Twain

FEAR is the acronym that we use to help your child manage all types of challenging situations. As you'll see, by teaching the FEAR plan, you'll be helping your child learn that there *is* a way to manage stress and negative emotions—a way to be in charge of how they feel. Although the meaning of the word *fear* is obviously applicable as an acronym to help manage anxiety, it was not chosen for that reason. Rather, each of the letters has a research basis for its usefulness as a step in the process of coping with stress and anxiety. The fact that the word *fear* also fits for managing anxiety came after the research findings and was somewhat serendipitous.

In this chapter, we provide a full overview of the FEAR plan and point out, along the way, how this helps your child not only manage emotion but also develop awareness, compassion, and resilience. To start, remember that you are a coach. A coach provides opportunities for someone to learn and practice new skills—skills that make you better at something. When we're in the parent role we often move too quickly to start problem solving and trying to make things easier, or we too quickly become frustrated, express our dissatisfaction, and give up. A coach knows there are a lot of fails and even some disappointments before skills start to develop, but these are not signs of disinterest or lack of effort; rather, they are the normal ups and downs of learning something new and challenging.

As you go through the FEAR plan, remember you'll have to put your own worries, frustrations, and deadlines on hold. Keep in mind also that *how* you communicate to your child can often be as important as *what* you communicate. Yelling or threatening doesn't work very well in getting kids to learn new things. All of us, both children and adults, learn much better when we are feeling relaxed—when we can be present. Be patient: Until you've gone through all the steps and your child has had several opportunities to practice, you can't expect to see them gain fluency. You are simply having important conversations and sharing valuable information that will build over time to create a lifetime of confidence and resilience.

Before we get into more specifics about how to teach the FEAR plan, let's first understand what makes up the acronym (and the plan).

The FEAR plan in a nutshell:

What Am I **F**eeling?

Expecting bad things to happen?

Attitudes and Actions that can help

Results and Rewards

F stands for "what am I **F**eeling?" The first step in managing anxiety is to identify it. First, we teach all about the physical symptoms of emotions. Your child will learn that their heart beating fast, butterflies in the stomach, headaches, and so on are all ways their body signals that there may be danger! Instead of worrying about these feelings, we see them as signs that an "alarm" is going off. But it may be a "*false* alarm." Now on to the next step of the FEAR plan.

E stands for "Expecting bad things to happen?" The second step is to ask yourself, *Am I expecting bad things to happen?* Here we pay attention to our thoughts. When we're feeling anxious, it's likely we're thinking about bad things that might happen. But are the thoughts accurate? Is there any other side to the story? Instead of going along with our first thought, we can make sure the thought we choose to go with is useful and accurate. Now on to the next step to decide what to do next.

A stands for "Attitudes and Actions that can help." With A, we put the FEA steps into action and approach the challenge. It's only when we approach a challenge, rather than try to avoid it, that we discover we are capable of handling difficult situations and emotions. We do this in a series of practices, sometimes called *exposures*, and through a lifestyle of approach. Now on to the last step of the FEAR plan.

R stands for "Results and Rewards." Kids (and parents) often set very high expectations and feel disappointed if things don't go exactly as they wanted. We remind them that they are still learning and growing. That no one is perfect. That, if they tried the F, E, and A steps, they can be proud and learn from the experience. The more they try, the easier it will get, and the more likely they'll have the outcome they hope for one day. The R step reminds them to reward themselves for their effort, not their outcomes. The reward will help them push when the effort feels hard and will also help them learn that doing things that are tough can be uncomfortable at first but feels really good in the end.

F Stands for What Am I Feeling?

The first step in managing anxiety is to identify it. How do you know when you are anxious? As we discussed in chapter 2, anxiety comes in a variety of physical, cognitive, and behavioral presentations. As an example, when one of your authors (PCK) gets anxious, I experience dry mouth and I start to notice and dwell on what I am thinking about. This *recursive thinking*, for me, is a sign of anxiety. Once you know your signs and experience of anxiety, these signs become cues for you to use your new skills. When I sense dry mouth, I pause. When I experience recursive thinking, it's a cue for me to speak what's on my mind, and to not overly rehearse it.

For the F step, you'll coach your child about the physical symptoms of anxiety—rapid heart beating, butterflies in the stomach, worrying, or even being jittery. They'll learn to figure out whether these reactions are a false alarm. Over time, our bodies can get in the habit of misreading physical signals and giving us alarms at the wrong times. It's our job to train our bodies to know when there is real danger and when there is no danger. We want to identify these feelings and to not be concerned about them. They are only signals that we need to evaluate as real or false alarms. Instead of worrying about these feelings, we go to the next step of the FEAR plan.

E Stands for Expecting Bad Things to Happen?

Once your child is comfortable recognizing their anxious arousal, they can ask themself, *Am I expecting bad things to happen?* In the E step of the FEAR plan, you'll coach your child on how to pay attention to inner thoughts (Expectations). Remember, we're all prone to thinking about all the unwanted things that might happen. When anxiety sneaks in, it likes to suggest that something bad might happen. Something bad might indeed happen, in some cases—it may be possible, but it is also very unlikely. You'll coach your child to identify when anxiety sneaks in and tries to take over; to recognize the thoughts and to not accept them at face value.

"Just because you think it, does not mean it will happen."

"Just because you think it, does not mean it is likely to happen."

Once your child has gained some skill in recognizing anxious thoughts and seeing them as only thoughts, the goal is for them to challenge the anxious thoughts with questions.

When a child thinks something bad will happen, we encourage them to challenge the initial thought and then choose the thought they have decided will be most accurate and most useful. To challenge the initial thought, they can ask questions like, "Are there other possibilities for what might happen?" Or, "What's usually happened in the past?" "What are some of the other sides to the story?" These questions help children collect evidence to support or refute their thoughts and build a repertoire of thoughts more focused on what they *do* have and what they *can* do—in other words, successful coping. Even when there is a problem that needs to be addressed, we practice developing independence and confidence in problem solving rather than focusing on the feeling of being overwhelmed.

Once you've addressed the two opening questions ("What are you *feeling?* and "Do you *expect* bad things to happen?"), it's time to go to the next step of the FEAR plan and begin to challenge, or practice approaching the situations that prompted these thoughts.

A Stands for Attitudes and Actions That Can Help

So far, we've learned that when an alarm goes off, you can remind yourself that it's a false alarm and it's time to think of a more accurate and more useful way to interpret the situation. In the A step of the FEAR plan, we decide on the attitude and the action that will best help us achieve our goal—that is, our chosen response. Again, when we are worried about an outcome, our first instinct is often to retreat or avoid the situation. If you've avoided or pushed away the negative feeling, you end up learning that things are really stressful and hard and you're not capable of handling them. The "bad" feeling will continue to arise in situations where there is challenge, and it could even gain strength over time. Until you do the thing you've put off or avoided, your mind and body won't really feel much better or learn anything new about these types of situations.

In the A step, we practice approaching (not avoiding) those situations that had been the source of distress. We help our kids create a plan to carry out a series of practices designed to implement the FEA steps, building up gradually from least difficult to most difficult situations, and then carry out and repeat the practices a few times. They learn from their own experience that they are capable of overcoming fears, disappointments, and challenges. Soon they won't need to practice; they'll have built up to a new level of confidence. At that point we continue to encourage a lifestyle of approach. As they accumulate experiences of being strong and competent, over time they develop self-confidence and resilience.

R Stands for Results and Rewards

In the R step, we review the results and reward the approaching challenges. This does not mean grading. Rather, it is reviewing what your child felt, what they thought, and what they did in trying the new or difficult thing, and then rewarding the process. Kids often set high expectations and then feel disappointed if things don't go exactly as they wanted. We encourage them to see that *trying* is the most important achievement by rewarding the trying (say, they applied for a summer job), not the outcome (they got the job, or didn't). It is a series of tries that leads to reaching a goal—so even a small and "unsuccessful" attempt is a move toward a goal, and every move toward the goal is rewarded. When they try, they can be proud that they did something challenging and learned from the experience.

Okay, we've completed our overview of the FEAR plan. The following chapters walk you step by step through the plan and how to communicate the plan to your child in full detail. Once you know the steps and feel comfortable with the content (so you're prepared to be the coach), you'll be ready to start sharing the FEAR plan with your child. For now, let's turn to some practical suggestions that will help you get started.

Key Takeaways

- F stands for What am I Feeling?

  The first step in managing anxiety is to identify it. Their heart beating fast, butterflies in the stomach, and headaches are some of the body's signals that there may be danger. Instead of worrying about these feelings, we see them as signs that an alarm is going off.

- E stands for Expecting bad things to happen?

  When we're feeling anxious, it's likely we're thinking about bad things that might happen. Instead of going along with our first thought, we can make sure the thought we choose to go with is useful and accurate.

- A stands for Attitudes and Actions that can help.

  It's only when we approach the challenge, rather than avoid it, that we discover that we are capable of handling difficult situations and emotions.

- R stands for Results and Rewards.

  The R step reminds kids to reward themselves for their effort, not for the outcomes. The reward will help them push when the effort feels hard and will also help them learn that doing things that are tough can be uncomfortable at first but feels really good in the end.

  To introduce the FEAR plan, find a time when there is calm—not in the middle of a struggle. Set appropriate expectations: managing emotions can come only after your child learns some skills and has plenty of practice.

CHAPTER 4

Your Role as Coach

A great coach can lead you to a place where you don't need him anymore.

—Andre Agassi

Before you start working with your child to help them with stress and anxiety, we want to give you some tips to set the stage for success. For starters, we recommend you start to think of yourself less as a parent and more as a coach.

There is great merit in being a coach who doesn't expect mastery from day 1, who creates opportunities for guided learning, and who rewards successful efforts without harsh criticism of errors. The best coaches act as mentors, using a calm, encouraging style. They use practice as opportunities to teach skills and a time for trying new skills, and to let players show what they have learned in the safe environment of a game. In this environment, players push themselves, take risks, and build self-confidence.

When we first became parents, it may have been the first time we fell into the role of caretaker. All of a sudden someone was depending on us for survival. We can all agree that we don't always know what's best, but we take on the role of someone who is all-knowing. We enact the role of an authority figure—a benevolent dictator of sorts.

Our own beliefs about what it means to be a parent come from, among many things, our memories of our own parents (our learning history), our interpretation of their parenting style, beliefs about our childhood, and messages communicated through our culture. These shape our behaviors and the emotions that follow. We anticipate threats to protect those we love, which again activates our overactive fight-or-flight response system, and we begin our own cycle of planning and preventing—anything to mitigate the threat. Too often, when we are in the role of parent, we react from fear. Instead of telling our kids to love, learn, grow, and give, we more often say things like "Watch out!" "You'll get left behind," or "The world is a dangerous place." We encourage risk aversion—which can also be referred to as fear. We teach them, from a very young age, to fear consequences and to fear authority. Imagine how much this can multiply over ten to twelve years. Needless to say, that is not the best point at which to begin developing one's ability to overcome adversity.

Awareness is the gift you can offer. You are not in a position to change your child's awareness directly, only to share your knowledge—to coach. Place your focus on the word *share* rather than *change*. You may have thought you had more control over your child than you do. Of course, you have great influence—the greatest influence—on your child. The words and actions you have shared, the experiences you created together, all have a profound influence on your child's understanding of themself and their world. But change doesn't come only from learning through observation and listening. Change comes as a result of their unique interpretation and emotional and physiological response to those experiences.

Remember, from CBT, that responses are shaped by their consequences. Now apply this to anxiety. Anxiety feels bad, so either (1) the removal of anxiety or (2) the perceived prevention of anxiety feels good initially. When an anxious teen skips a day of school and believes that this prevents an embarrassing situation, then the teen will be more likely to again skip a day of school. Our behaviors and our children's behaviors are increased, decreased, or shaped by the consequences of the behavior.

Good coaching involves being aware of the behaviors and consequences that are reinforcing or maintaining the anxiety that your child experiences. It is important to: (1) become expert in knowing the behaviors, antecedents, and consequences associated with your child's anxiety, and (2) be aware and in control of your own behaviors, especially your reactions to your child's anxiety or anxious behaviors.

To share these concepts, it will be important to first practice applying these principles to yourself. Practice awareness of what you feel, physically and emotionally. Step back. Practice having a conversation with yourself. Become aware of the thought preceding the feeling, then go back further to becoming aware of the stories or beliefs that underlie the thought. This requires letting go of many rules and learnings. It is time to be deliberate. When you don't feel good, it is the start of a process, a conversation that must be had. *I am aware of the emotion I'm feeling. Where did this come from? What did I just say to myself that made me feel this way? Do I believe it? How long do I want to accept feeling this way? What do I really believe? What do I really know about this? I'm not asking someone else to do something or to change—what is it that I need to think and do to feel how I want?*

It's no longer a matter of what you *thought* you need, but knowing what you really want, and doing what you truly intend. It will have nothing to do with anyone or anything else. You'll be working toward consistently showing that you stand in love and appreciation of your true meaning, your true purpose. Sticking with this new idea, even an unpopular new idea, requires a paradigm shift. When you make a decision to do this, you have made a decision to give your child the gift of freedom to pursue.

Become an Expert on Your Child's Anxiety

Don't rush into trying to make big changes. Before starting to try to make any changes, know when your child's anxiety is most likely be expressed, what it looks like in your child, and what usually happens next. It takes time to gather this information: before you try and make changes like a coach, watch and learn your child's habits, skills, and challenges. It takes time to gather this information, but it will not only help make the anxiety feel more predictable (to both you and your child), but also will play a key role in successfully reducing the anxiety. When your child's anxiety becomes predictable, it will feel less overwhelming to you.

Anxiety usually follows a pattern, and this is very likely true for your child. The pattern makes it predictable in many ways. We often explain to parents that "your brain has figured out what it can get your attention with." Although we don't mean for this statement to be taken literally, it communicates an important notion well. Consider yourself as an example: you may have noticed that you get particularly anxious in social situations at work. Your brain increasingly attends to negative outcomes in these situations: you may think to yourself, *I may say something that doesn't sound smart,* so you hold back and, over time, become increasingly uncomfortable every time you're in a social situation at work. As a consequence, you may build up a pattern of behavior. Perhaps you overprepare for presentations, avoid social activities at work, or steer away from tasks that would put you in the spotlight.

Knowing your pattern is useful. Using this example, the next time you have a social engagement at work coming up, you'll know in advance that your anxiety will increase; you'll know what it will feel like and what will probably happen next. You can feel less upset when it comes (you knew it was coming) and you may even decide to do something differently. Similarly, it will be very useful for you to know more about the pattern of your child's anxiety.

There may be multiple situations that provoke anxiety for your child. Select just one for your initial effort to answer the questions in the "Ask yourself" boxes. Therapists refer to this process as a *functional analysis* because it helps identify the function of a behavior. After you have had a chance to think it through, and even a chance to revise what you thought, you can apply the same process to other situations. Work through all the steps for each situation. Don't expect to be an expert, and don't expect to discover anything magical. Indeed, it is possible you won't know exactly what your child's anxiety is about, but you'll improve your understanding of the situations that trigger your child's anxiety, how your child responds, and the difficult behaviors associated with the anxious responding. Try to identify the purpose that the behavior is serving and what is maintaining the behavior.

Ask yourself:

1. In what situations do you notice that anxiety typically arises for your child?

2. What does it typically look like, both the outward manifestations and your child's description of how they feel?

3. What behaviors does your child exhibit when anxious?

4. What usually happens next?

5. What are some things your child tries to help relieve anxiety?

6. What are the typical results or consequences of these efforts?

Know your reaction to your child's anxiety—and be in control of it.

Ask yourself:

1. What do you usually do when you notice your child being anxious?

2. What do you usually do when you anticipate an anxiety-provoking situation?

3. What usually happens next?

4. What are some strategies you have given your child to help them relieve their anxiety?

5. What are the typical results or consequences of these strategies?

6. What usually happens next?

7. Is your reaction reinforcing the behavior or weakening it?

8. Would you choose to react differently or add anything to what you are currently doing?

Again, as a parent you are an important role model for how to react to different situations. Your reactions will shape your child's future behavior. And this includes both reinforcing certain behaviors—making it occur more frequently—and not reinforcing other behaviors so they fade away over time. For instance, if your daughter makes an effort to talk to those "popular" kids who scare her, and it goes fine, and you acknowledge this, that might encourage her to attend school more often. And if talking to those kids ends up sending her into an anxiety cycle, and you don't reinforce that anxiety by trying to assuage it, but instead guide her to navigate the anxiety she's feeling, that might encourage her to be less susceptible to her anxiety in the future.

A large part of responding in this adaptive way—of being your child's anxiety coach, as much as you're her parent—is about the second principle of shaping: responding to her anxiety in ways in line with your values, rather than acting on your fears.

Convey Your Values, Not Your Fears

Your reaction to your child's anxiety is an important response to be aware of, but equally as important is your reaction to the situation. Do you find yourself worried that they might not make the team or cast of the play? Worried about their grades in school? Worried they may not have enough friends? Worried they might not get enough sleep? Some parents even worry, when the child is only ten or eleven, about whether they will get into a preferred college. If you find yourself feeling anxious about the situation, even if you do not intend to be, this will impact how you respond to your child's anxiety.

Will you feel anxious? Of course you will. Can your anxiety be justified? Of course it can. What parent wouldn't want to see their child make the team or the school play, be able to give a quality book report, or come home with an impressive report card? What parent wouldn't hope to see their child be accepted into a preferred college? But a parent's response to these important milestones often reveals their greatest personal strengths and weaknesses. And when a parent responds with fear, it's not the most helpful response. As part of helping with your child's anxiety, it's time to consider your own emotional control, your own pride, and your own display of anxiety.

Think for a moment: What do you do when your child expresses or displays anxiety? You might find yourself quick to react, short-tempered, and impatient. That has clear disadvantages when it comes to addressing a child's anxiety. Or you may find that you are the opposite—overly empathetic, eager to solve the problem or be the person to relieve the stress. Stepping in quickly to reduce the child's anxiety, although it may come from a desire to be a good parent, communicates to the child that they can't handle it themself. When a parent steps in, this can communicate to the child, even if unwittingly, that they can't handle the situation but instead need the parent to solve it for them. Although each specific situation and child has distinct circumstances and nuances, it is important to remember that it is not the single win or loss in a game, the one grade in one class, or the name of the college; rather, it is about the development of skills for handling emotions and distress, for learning, growing, and persevering.

Ask yourself:

1. What are your beliefs, experiences, and values about anxiety that influence your response?

2. What are your fears about your child's situation?

3. How will you handle an outcome that you are afraid of (such as not winning a game, getting a bad SAT score, or missing an important event)?

4. Has your belief and/or fear influenced your response to your child?

5. What is it that you want your child to learn from this experience, and what needs to happen for them to learn it? (Try defining your idea of "success" for your child.)

Not Parenting, But Coaching

A coach teaches skills that help a child get better at a task or skill, whereas a parent might try to make things better for them. In this section, we'll explore some skills that will help you make the shift from parent to coach so you can really help your child confront their anxiety: deal with the feelings of fear and worry they might be feeling, challenge the worries that are keeping them stuck, and discover that they *can* actually deal with them.

Be confident: They will get there. Your belief about whether your child can or can't handle a difficult situation absolutely gets communicated in your interactions with them. When your child "reads" your beliefs, they will act from it (you've likely experienced when your child falls, then looks to your reaction, and starts crying when they see that you're worried).

This is why it is so important for you to know and truly believe that the situation is something he will be able to handle.

If your son said he wasn't sure he would ever be able to do multiplication, you wouldn't be worried or communicate that you were worried that maybe he wouldn't. You'd want to communicate your strong belief that it can be hard at first but that he'll practice a little every day and eventually will get it. Similarly, you wouldn't give up and say "Okay, you don't ever have to learn multiplication"—you'd just find smaller steps and different ways to teach, and urge him to keep practicing. That's the same with anxiety—you can find smaller steps, different ways to practice, but you must keep practicing—there's no such thing as "can't," just "haven't yet." Know for sure that he will get there.

If parents were asking the teacher for an accommodation to write a book report instead of read it in front of class, or let the child miss school on presentation day, they would be relieving anxiety temporarily, but then reinforcing the child's learning that there really was danger, and they weren't able to handle it.

Be patient: A seasoned coach doesn't feel frustrated if it takes a few tries for the child to become more confident with a new skill.

As you go through the steps, remember you'll have to put your worries, frustrations, and deadlines on hold. Your child will be learning a new skill. Until you've gone through all the steps and they've had several opportunities to practice, you can't expect to see a great deal of change.

Realize that this can be hard for them at first, but if you are consistent with your message and actions each day, they will get there. They will see that you believe that it's important, and that they can do it. Then stay calm and steady in your plan, every time. Be careful not to ask "Do you think you'll be able to?" This communicates that you're not sure they can handle it.

You are on the same team: You are all fighting the worries—not each other. When we talk about worries, it often seems that arguments and frustrations are sparked. It might be that you've gotten into a you versus us pattern. *You* (your child) is too anxious and it seems to *us* (parents) that you should try to stop. A colleague and eminent researcher, Dr. John March, always recommended externalizing the anxiety—giving it a name or other identifying term—so you're not challenging your child; rather, you are both challenging, say, "the Bully."

Keep the praise-to-criticism ratio high (shoot for 5:1): Even when you know your child could do better with some effort, rather than first pointing out the mistakes, point out what they did well. Think in terms of improvement ("What were you working on this week?"), not perfection. Praise all good aspects of their resilience journey—not just that they were ultimately able to successfully overcome the challenge, but that along the way they have been thoughtful, helpful, supportive, funny, responsible, a good friend, and so on. Praise *during* the process, not after the outcome—this reinforces that process is what is valued. Praise persistence, problem-solving, creativity, teamwork, purpose—praise getting better at these, not achieving a specific outcome. Praise failure, too! "So great you tried this really hard thing." "You worked so hard; you're getting closer every time."

Listen, then wait, then listen some more: It is important to hear and acknowledge your child's worries as valid. If you are too quick to dismiss or invalidate the anxiety, your child may not trust that you understand or are taking them seriously. This hurts your ability to work as a team and might shut off honest and open communication.

Manage Your Own Anxiety

You may have heard before how important it is to model the types of behaviors you want to see in your child. Modeling is a central principle in CBT approaches. Children are learning about the world and how to respond to it by watching how *you* see the world and how you respond. Over time, your modeled behavior, including how you handle stress and challenges, shapes how your child learns to handle stress and challenges.

If you find yourself reacting to your own stress with panic, anger, withdrawal, or avoidance, it's likely that your child will see this and use their own version of similar reactions (such as panic and avoidance) when dealing with their own stresses. If you watch the news and hear a story about a toy recall and then decide that you and your kids should avoid certain types of toys and repeatedly remind them of toy manufacturer warnings, it's possible that your child will later develop discomfort with the thought of being harmed by certain types of toys or toys that have not been checked and preapproved by you. Over time this can build a pattern of avoidance and vulnerability in a "dangerous" world. Caution, when warranted, is wise; excessive checking and avoidance communicate the need for excessive worry.

Researchers have studied the overlaps in parental anxiety and child anxiety. One review of data on parents of anxious youth found that most studies reported from 60 to 80 percent of parents also had similar symptoms of anxiety. If you struggle with anxiety, you are not alone. Over 15 percent of the population will struggle with impairing anxiety in their lifetime, and many more with distressing anxiety. Research has also found a reciprocal relationship between parent and child anxiety: as one improves, there is improvement in the other!

The classic airplane analogy (put on your own oxygen mask before helping your child put theirs on) applies here. We must take care of ourselves before we can take care of anyone else. We create the feeling and emotion in our homes—when we are calm, home is calm; when we are stressed, our children feel stressed. We could spend this entire book describing tips for managing your own anxiety, but instead we'll direct you to a book on the topic—Tamar Chansky's *Freeing Yourself from Anxiety* (2012) and recommend that you reach out to your doctor or therapist to discuss if you feel you could benefit from consultation.

Keep It Fun

This is important: try to make the time you are working on this together very positive and fun! Keep an upbeat tone while you're explaining new concepts and practicing. Collaboration is key: it should feel like you're working on a project together.

One way to help keep it fun is to take a minute to think of some of your child's strengths (instead of only thinking about their worries) that will be helpful to them through this process. For example, some kids are creative; others have a sense of humor; still others may be musical. Think of some of their interests; computer games, movie characters, books. Keep these in mind when thinking of ways to explain and practice managing anxiety—bringing in themes and stories that are interesting and fun to your child will help them understand and remember what you're talking about.

Choose the Right Time to Talk

It is extremely important to time your discussions appropriately. It's very tempting to want to address a problem *now*. It may seem you don't want to lose the moment when the situation arises. But there are good reasons not to launch into a talk as soon as you get home from the party—"Let's talk about why you didn't say hello to anyone." In the immediate aftermath, anxiety is still high. Your child is likely to be distressed or reflecting on the discomfort they just experienced. Think of times when you've felt uncomfortable or bad about a recent situation: this is not when we're at our best for problem solving or thinking about how to approach things differently. We are still seeking relief from the bad feelings. Instead, try to wait until the bad feeling passes before starting to address difficult challenges.

When your child is anxious, or in the middle of an activity, is not the time. Have the conversation when they are feeling calm and able to focus for a few minutes.

Now you're ready to get started.

Key Takeaways

Before starting to share the FEAR plan with your child, be clear about the behaviors and consequences that are reinforcing or maintaining the anxiety that your child experiences:

- Become well versed in the behaviors, antecedents, and consequences associated with your child's anxiety.

- Be aware of and in control of your own behaviors, especially your reactions to your child's distress or avoidant behaviors.

Good coaching involves:

- Being confident in your child's ability to cope.

- Being patient—it will take time to develop and practice coping skills.

- Remembering that you are on the same team. Don't blame anyone or point out weaknesses; it's the anxiety "bully" that everyone is angry at, not each other.

- Keeping praise frequent and criticism specific and rare. Encourage behaviors and attitudes you'd want to see your child use more, and ignore the ones you want to see less.

- Listening, waiting, and then listening some more. Let them have their time to feel heard, to explain their experience and emotions. Wait before jumping in to correct them or start to problem solve—when you do that, it cuts off open communication and the potential for your child to develop their own self-confidence.

- Managing your own emotions. If you are stressed, it will be difficult to help them with their stress. Put self-care and structures of support in place for yourself before starting to work on the FEAR plan for your child.

- Keeping it fun. As a coach, you want to make their experience of learning and trying fun and rewarding.

PART 2

The Recipe

CHAPTER 5

The F Step: What Am I Feeling?

The physical symptoms of fight or flight are what the human body has learned over thousands of years to operate efficiently and at the highest level...anxiety is a cognitive interpretation of that physical response.

—John Eliot

Whether your child is stressed and down or is doing well and you're just hoping to give them the tools they'll need to live life with calmness and confidence, introducing them to the language of emotions will be invaluable. By gaining awareness of what they are feeling and how their body is responding, your child will also gain clarity and control over what they choose to do next. We might assume that this understanding comes naturally over time. And with cognitive development and life experience, kids do become more versed in understanding their emotions. But today, with less face-to-face social interaction and less time talking about feelings with parents and family members, kids may be missing out on developing the language and understanding of emotion. They might not be getting enough practice catching the clues of verbal and nonverbal communication or learning how to modulate their feelings—from mild to intense—in a way that will work for them in a range of situations. In addition, kids now can express their emotions online or via text message to large groups—settings in which developmentally normal missteps in emotion regulation and communication are subject to the comments, reactions, and pitiless judgments of a wider audience—well before they've developed a strong understanding of their emotions and how to communicate them. They may be more likely to suffer difficult consequences of large-scale rejection, confusion, and loneliness at a younger age.

It's a good idea to have these conversations sooner rather than later.

Bringing the FEAR Plan into a Conversation

Pick the right time to introduce the topic and initiate a conversation with your child—*not* when your child is feeling anxious or is in the middle of an activity. Have the conversation when your child is feeling calm, unburdened, and able to focus for a few minutes.

You can start by acknowledging that everyone feels sad, stressed, and anxious at times. That you know how it feels to be sad or really stressed and anxious. You can remind them that all feelings are normal and even negative emotions have a purpose—they can be great illuminators of what we care most about. Like if your pet has just died, it's not a time to feel happy. Your sadness shows how much your pet meant to you, the joy they gave you, and the love you felt. Over time, the sadness can teach us that loss is difficult, but temporary. When you realize the love, loyalty, and friendship you experienced, you feel a sense of peace— that you loved genuinely and unconditionally.

But there are times we feel more anxious or sad than we need to, or for too long, and it gets in the way and stops us from doing things we want to do or from focusing on the things that truly matter. You can then give an example of how anxiety may have been a block for you, getting in the way of something you really wanted to do, or taking too much energy and attention. You can then describe a time when it looked to you like anxiety got in the way of something your child really wanted to do—like learn something new or make a new friend.

Although we expect you will have your own way of successfully communicating with your child, and we don't mean to dictate a specific set of words, we offer suggested conversation starters to help guide you in moving the conversation forward.

CONVERSATION STARTER Everyone feels stressed and sad sometimes. People worry. Do you know what it feels like to feel anxious or stressed? Sadness and anxiety are normal. They are emotions we all feel at times. Sometimes these are useful. But there are times when we feel more anxious or sad than we need to. It's tough being a kid these days—between school, homework, grades, friends, sports, it's no wonder you're stressed out once in a while. Sometimes the negative feelings get in the way and stop us from doing things we want to do, or we stay feeling bad for too long. But it doesn't have to be stronger than we are. There are things we can do to be more in control of anxiety and of how we feel in general.

I want to teach you the FEAR plan. It was created by scientists [that is, it's not just your own ideas about what will help], and it works really well to help people manage their stress and worry and feel better. The FEAR plan is great because it helps not only in situations that make you nervous, but in all kinds of stressful situations. And once you know how to use it, you'll be able to help yourself feel better when you're feeling more worried or sad than you want to be. The four steps of the plan start with the letters F, E, A, and R, which makes it easy to remember the steps. Each week for the next few weeks, we'll go over one of the steps. Once you've got the hang of it, we'll practice using the plan. We'll start with easy practices and then try some challenging ones—the more we do, the easier it will get.

The F Step: What Am I Feeling?

The first step in managing emotions is to identify them. The F step in the FEAR plan reminds them to do just that—recognize and label what they are feeling and understand the physiological process behind the emotion. This slows down the automatic reaction:

Situation ➔ Response

and moves them to

Situation ➔ Recognize Physiological and Emotional Reaction

putting your child in a position to think through their chosen response.

When you introduce the F step, you'll be explaining that emotions often come and go, and we usually don't think too much about it—it feels like there's not much we can do about what we are feeling. But there is actually a lot we can do! We are in charge of how we are feeling—but first we have to recognize our feelings. That's the focus of the F step.

CONVERSATION STARTER   We may say, "I'm sad' or "I'm nervous" but not really think about it much more than that. We just go with the feeling and feel like there's nothing we can do about it. But there is something we can do to have control over how we feel. As soon as we notice a "big" or "bad" feeling, it's our cue to use the FEAR plan. The letters F-E-A-R will walk us through the steps to feeling better.

The first step, the F step, reminds us that the first thing we have to do is to stop and notice the feeling and then give it a name. In the F step, we ask ourself *What am I **F**eeling?* and then decide what word we'd use to describe the feeling. We don't have to just let feelings come and go—we want to know exactly what we are feeling so that we can be in a good position to know what we want to do next.

Though it may be tempting, try not to bring this up after your child has a meltdown or crying spell or after a big argument with a sibling or friend. As we mentioned in the previous chapter, it's more likely to be effective if you plan for a few minutes at the end of the day to discuss this, rather than trying to teach it when a big emotion has appeared: first, because it communicates that you both are working on something important together, and second, because it's not usually effective to try to teach new things when they are focused on something else.

Identifying Emotions

Kids learn the common feeling words, like happy, sad, excited, and angry, fairly early on but aren't as proficient with some of the more specific emotion words, like disappointed, hurt, anxious, lonely, or frustrated. We want to *expand their range and depth of understanding of emotions.* We recommend starting with a conversation or activity by listing as many feeling words as you and your child can think of and then discussing what the feeling "looks" like and feels like.

Sample beginning: "To be able to make the F step really work, we'll have to get really good at knowing what we are feeling, what feelings look like, and where they come from."

Take a moment to *normalize having a range of emotions.* Share a story about when you had a negative feeling—a story that you're confident your child is developmentally ready and able to understand. Your sharing helps normalize different emotions and conveys that we all have ups and downs in our emotions.

Sample: "I experience bad feelings too, and you've seen me have a 'big' feeling before! Do you remember the time..."

Spend some time discussing why you would choose that feeling word rather than another (say, annoyed versus frustrated, bored versus lonely, worried versus scared).

Also *point out that different feelings have different physical expressions and facial expressions,* which can be clues to how we are feeling.

"How can we tell, besides from what they are saying, if someone is worried, angry, sad, or happy? Right: their facial expression and even the way their body looks really tells us a lot about how they're feeling."

Here are some other ideas for how to have this conversation:

- **Play "Feelings Charades"**—Take turns picking a feeling word to act out without using words; the other guesses the feeling just by the facial expression and body posture. This points out non-verbal cues and clues for different emotions and increases your child's awareness about these. For each feeling, think of a situation you would have liked to act out if you were able to use words—a good way to learn what your child knows and understands about these words and an opportunity to fill in the gaps if you hear any. For example, if your child acts out the feeling of *frustrated* by acting really angry, and their story is that they didn't get the toy they wanted, you could suggest that there is another word that is good for times when things don't turn out how you hoped: *disappointed*. Disappointed looks less angry and more sad, but not necessarily crying, because in this case it was just a small disappointment of not getting a toy they were looking forward to getting, not a big disappointment like learning that your good friend is moving to another state. You could add that frustrated is great to describe when you keep trying something and no matter how hard you try, it just doesn't seem to work—like a science fair project that keeps falling apart.

- **Create a Feelings Dictionary**—In magazines or online, find pictures of people showing different expressions, both facial and entire body, that reflect different emotions. Discuss what type of feeling each person is experiencing. Cut out or print out the photos and put them on construction paper with a caption labeling each emotion.

- **Play Feelings Hangman**—Take turns picking an *uncommon* feeling word for the other person to guess. After the correct word is revealed, discuss what the feeling looks like, when it comes up, and whether they can recall any situations where they felt that way.

Notice that in the suggestions we've stayed general and didn't recommend focusing on a specific emotion that your child is struggling with. We first want to keep the conversation open and not make your child feel put on the spot to share things that either are difficult or embarrassing or could make them feel criticized or convey that they have done something wrong. We want to convey the opposite: that all feelings are normal, and we all feel them. Especially because this will be one of the first conversations you have about managing emotions and the FEAR plan with your child, you want it to be associated with good feelings and fun so they will feel comfortable talking and sharing with you moving forward.

In general, we recommend practicing "using the right word" as you are going about your days. If you notice a feeling of your own, name it out loud. If you notice your child feeling something, either negative or positive, you can ask "What word would you pick for how you're feeling?" or remind them, "Wait—make sure you're using the right word for that feeling—it might change what you decide to do next."

It Might Be a False Alarm!

It's natural for our body to feel more tired and lethargic when we are down. We can have stomachaches when we are stressed. These are called *somatic symptoms* of the emotion—or, physical symptoms. Somatic symptoms of different emotions can be surprising and sometimes upsetting. For example, dizziness, shortness of breath, insomnia, fatigue, or diarrhea can all happen when we are anxious or down. Sometimes the symptoms themselves can cause anxiety or low mood. For instance, worrying about not being able to sleep can increase anxiety, which can make it more difficult to get to sleep. Gaining a good understanding of physiological processes can help your child feel less surprised or upset by any physical symptom and feel more in control—and this may reduce their worry or stress about the symptoms themselves. Kids often have difficulty making the connection between physical symptoms of anxiety and anxiety-provoking events. For example, when a child who feels sick before a spelling test or sports, their body might be giving them a clue or warning sign that they are feeling worried.

An important part of teaching the F step is teaching your child about our body's built-in alarm system—the fight-or-flight response. Kids who tend to be more anxious can have sensitive alarms. When they are in a difficult situation, they may feel lots of uncomfortable physical sensations. Their stomach might hurt, their heart might race, they might feel a headache or nausea. Rather than worrying about these sensations, we want them to know that's just their body's way of telling them they're feeling a little frightened. Kids who are not necessarily sensitive will also have a natural fight-or-flight response to challenges or uncertainty from time to time. Even they will benefit from knowing what's happening inside their bodies and why.

CONVERSATION STARTER   It's really amazing, actually—our body is designed to protect us from danger. If we were in the forest being chased by a bear, our built-in alarm system would automatically go to work to put our body into action to do what we need to do—either stay and "fight" (if we want to punch the bear in the nose), or take "flight" (get away as fast as we can to outrun the bear), or "freeze" (hide and stay still so the bear doesn't spot us). That's why some people call it the "fight, flight, or freeze" response. Once our system senses danger, the alarm goes off, and all of these changes start taking place in your body—including making your heart race (to pump blood to your muscles), making your muscles tense (so you can fight hard or run really fast), and making you take shorter, faster breaths (so you can get oxygen to your muscles to help you be fast and strong). It's usually not time to eat a sandwich when there's a bear chasing after you, so your body knows to pause the digestive system as well. This is why, when we are anxious, we sometimes feel tummy aches or butterflies or have to run to use the bathroom!

Can you think of a time when you experienced a fight, flight, or freeze response?

Let them describe their different experiences with fight or flight. You can give examples of a time it happened to you.

It usually works beautifully—it stops us from crossing the road if we hear a car coming, or makes us duck before the ball hits us in the nose. And it does all of this automatically. We don't need to decide to do anything. But sometimes the alarm goes off too often. It thinks too many things are dangerous. Your body's alarm might go off any time there's something new or different, or that might be different from what you're used to, or that could be difficult or embarrassing. Worrying is actually part of your body's alarm system too—it's your brain trying to give you ideas about what you should do about the dangers that might be out there. If it keeps going off whenever there is a new or difficult situation, it can be really uncomfortable and make you feel like you're not going to be okay.

It's our job to teach our brain that we are not in danger—we do that by recognizing the signs of a fight-or-flight response. When we know the signs, we don't have to react as strongly or feel worried about them. We know it's just a false alarm and that we have to teach our brain that we are uncomfortable because we are doing something new or challenging, but we are not in danger.

"The fire trucks can go home! I'm just worried about something!"

You sometimes tell me you have a stomachache before a test. That's an example—your fight-or-flight system has gone off at the wrong time. It sensed you were worried about something, and the alarm went off! Your body shuts off blood to your stomach because it's preparing to run (not to eat!) and so your stomach gets queasy.

The first step in worrying less (or teaching your body that there's no bear sneaking up behind you) is to know what your body feels like when the alarm goes off.

What happens in your body when one of these things happens?

- You hear a noise in the middle of the night.

- You see a scary part in a movie.

- You have to answer a question out loud in class.

- You have to perform in a recital or a big game or competition.

What else do you feel when you get nervous or tense? These feelings are all part of your body's alarm system. The system starts your heart beating fast and speeds up your breathing to get air and blood to your muscles so you can *run!*

This is going to be really helpful, because now every time you notice one of these feelings, you'll know that you must be feeling worried or anxious. Instead of worrying about these feelings, I want you to just notice them. Once you notice them pop up, you've just gotten through the first step of the FEAR plan. You ask yourself, *What am I Feeling?* and if you notice any of those symptoms, the answer might be *I'm feeling nervous, and my body's alarm has gone off when it didn't need to.*

Body Map Activity

On a blank piece of paper, draw an outline of a body (don't worry about your artistic talent—it's okay if it looks like a funky gingerbread man). Have your child draw what happens in their body when they are feeling sad, anxious, excited, or angry.

Alternatively, have them choose their physical symptoms they recognize on this list:

Fast heartbeat	Stomachache
Pounding heart	Trouble sleeping
Fast breathing	Trembling or shakiness
Blushing	Tired
Dizziness	Headache
Shortness of breath	Sweating or feeling warm
Butterflies	Restlessness
Nausea	Difficulty concentrating
Muscle tension	Aches, pains

These feelings will be your clues or signal to know it's time to use the FEAR plan to help yourself feel more calm and in control. We're going to learn these strategies together.

This is a perfect time to point out that over time, our body forms habits. So we're not necessarily reacting physically to a new challenge or an anticipated problem; we may just be having a physical response out of habit!

CONVERSATION STARTER You'll probably see that the same physical feelings come again and again around the same time or in the same types of situations. It's helpful to spot your pattern because then you won't feel as surprised or worried the next time it comes up. It also gives you a chance to change something if you don't like the pattern you are in.

During the next few days, pay attention to your body's alarm system. On paper or in a journal, write down if that alarm goes off. Then describe how it makes your body feel.

Let's see if we can find any patterns.

- My alarm went off when: [possibilities: when I woke up, before English class, before soccer practice, on my way to school]

- My body felt: [possibilities: heart beating fast, tired, stomachache]

These are the situations when your body shows you that you're nervous or that you're worrying too much. Your body's alarm is in the habit of going off in the same types of situations. It's helpful to spot your alarm pattern, because then you won't feel as surprised or worried the next time it comes up. It also gives you a chance to change something if you don't like the pattern you are in. Your alarm will tell you *Don't do it! You're not okay! Lie down instead!* That's the time to remind your body that it's just sounding a false alarm. Say to yourself, *I'm not in danger; I'm just worried.* Then it will be time to move to the next step of the FEAR plan.

Key Takeaways (For You and Your Child)

Normalizing negative emotions helps make it safe, not embarrassing or overwhelming, to feel down or anxious.

Expanding your child's breadth and depth of understanding different emotions will give them more awareness of their own experience and opens more options for deciding what they choose to do next.

The F step in the FEAR plan reminds them to recognize and label what they are feeling and understand the physiological process behind the emotion.

Rather than worrying about these sensations, we want them to know that these are just their body's way of telling them they're anxious or anticipating something negative.

They learn about the "fight, flight, or freeze" response and that sometimes we might feel the symptoms of the response (breathing fast, heart beating fast, nausea, and so on). Sometimes our brain makes a mistake: it was a false alarm; we were just doing something that is new or difficult, not dangerous.

It is our job to teach our brain that we are not in danger—we do this by recognizing that it's a false alarm and then moving to the next step of the FEAR plan.

CHAPTER 6

Relaxation Training, Meditation, and Mindfulness

If you are quiet enough, you will hear the flow of the universe. You will feel its rhythm. Go with this flow. Happiness lies ahead. Meditation is key.

—Buddha

Our kids today, as early as they are born, are overstimulated with the sounds of technology, "learning toys," and television. As they grow, this is combined with a multitude of activities, requirements, and pressure from schools and parents to "hurry up." In general, a mind that is encouraged to learn and be challenged is a good thing. But being able to calm our mind and body is an extremely important piece of what is needed to be able to grow.

When we think of ways to reset and relax, many of us look for places to go or activities to do. We plan to go to the beach, read a book, or take a warm bath. Certainly those things can be relaxing, but we shouldn't need a beach in order to feel calm. In fact, when we create plans like going to the beach or taking a warm bath, they are often planned as escapes from our everyday stresses. As we've learned, escapes are only temporarily relieving and can create more stress and anxiety in the long term. Planning an escape sends our body the message that where and how we are is not okay—that it's time to flee. So we want help our kids know how to be relaxed *without* going to the beach or anywhere else. Here's how.

Relaxation Training

Relaxation training is an integral part of helping kids (and adults) reset and increase resilience to stress and anxiety and even depressed mood. It has many proven benefits, including eased muscle tension, reduced worry, improved concentration, and better sleep. Relaxation training includes techniques such as progressive muscle relaxation, breathing training, and visualization. It works by sending the message to the nervous system that there is no danger, that you are safe. As we have learned, when the fight-or-flight system kicks in, it very quickly and automatically starts a physiological process that speeds up heart rate and breathing, muscle readiness, increased blood circulation, and hormone release—putting us in heightened arousal and panic mode. This stress response is not helpful when the danger is not real and we're trying to stay in control. When we guide our body to breathe deeply and relax our muscles slowly, it sends the message to our brain that we are not in danger. This helps shut down the false alarm and get us back to feeling calm and in control. Doing a form of relaxation every day for a few weeks helps build up our reserves to stay in a more relaxed state and makes it even easier and faster to send the "everything is okay" message to our brain.

Here we describe three effective and easy relaxation techniques: diaphragmatic breathing, progressive muscle relaxation, and guided imagery. Try all of the methods together, then let your child decide which one they like best, or choose to practice a combination. We'll describe each and give you some ways to help your child learn. We have included language that can be helpful for children, but feel free to make changes to fit your child best.

Technique 1: Diaphragmatic Breathing

Children who are experiencing high levels of stress and anxiety tend to breathe shallowly, taking short breaths only into their chest. Shallow breathing creates an imbalance of oxygen and carbon dioxide, which can lead to lightheadedness, tingling, chest pain, and other sensations that can be felt as anxiety. In fact, some kids get stuck in a worry cycle, worrying about these uncomfortable feelings; some can even escalate into panic from these internal sensations.

Diaphragmatic breathing, also known as *belly breathing*, is a natural way of breathing—it's how we breathe when we are born. As we grow, we tend to rush our breathing and start to center our breathing in our chest. Diaphragmatic breathing is a relaxation technique that helps your child slow down their breathing and use the diaphragm correctly while doing so. It helps to (1) improve focus on breathing rather than negative thoughts, (2) decrease the work of breathing by slowing their breathing rate, and (3) decrease oxygen demand. They then use less effort and energy to breathe, sending the message to their brain that there is no danger. It's easy to do:

1. Pretend your stomach is a balloon that you're trying to blow up. Breathe deeply into your stomach (blow up the balloon, counting in your mind to 5).

2. Exhale completely, through your mouth, blowing all the air out of the balloon until it's empty (again counting to 5).

3. Repeat for three minutes, imagining all the air going all through your body through every muscle, from your head to your toes.

Diaphragmatic breathing uses the diaphragm muscle located under our ribs and above our abdomen. When we breathe in, we push the muscle down, and our tummy is pushed forward. When we breathe out, the diaphragm rises back to its resting position and our tummy flattens. There is little or no upper chest movement.

Before becoming the coach for your child, first learn for yourself how to engage in diaphragmatic breathing. Try to swell out your belly as you fill your lungs deeply with air, like you would when you are blowing up a balloon. Now slowly let out all the air, like you're trying to blow out a candle. Breathe in through your nose (count 1 and 2), and out through your mouth (count 1 and 2). We suggest that you practice once or twice each day, and soon you'll have it. With this simple change in your breathing you can bring on relaxation. And you can do it without anyone noticing.

Encourage your child to find a comfortable position to sit and pay attention to their breathing. Ask them to place a hand on their belly to feel it filling and emptying and follow along with you. A friendly reminder: be a collaborating coach. Patience and cooperation pave the road to relaxation.

Your child now has the deep breathing strategy to use as a tool whenever they need to feel calm.

Technique 2: Progressive Muscle Relaxation

We can learn to induce deep muscular relaxation by tensing and then releasing tension from various parts of the body, one part at a time. This is highly effective in signaling to your brain that everything is okay. By tensing and then releasing, we also learn to differentiate between tense and relaxed muscles. To provide a firsthand experience, the following is a script-like description of the process of progressive muscle relaxation. You can use it yourself first, then adapt it to be used with your child. First there is breathing, then there is the tense-and-relax pairing.

The overall goal is to tense all of the muscle groups in your body for four to eight seconds and then relax the muscle groups, one at a time, in order from head to toes, all while slowing your breathing and focusing on the muscles. You can sit in a chair or lie down while doing this.

1. Slow breathing:

   I want you to take a slow deep breath to the count of 5 (*count in seconds*), 1-2-3-4-5, and let it out, 1-2-3-4-5.

   Breathe again, in through your nose, 1-2-3-4-5, and out through your mouth, 1-2-3-4-5. One more time, take a deep breath, make sure your belly gets really big and you fill up your lungs—like you're blowing up a balloon in your tummy. Good, now let it out, 1-2-3-4-5. Again, breathe in, 1-2-3-4-5, and exhale, 1-2-3-4-5.

2. Hands:

Now, take your right hand and pretend you're holding a lemon and trying to squeeze out all the juice. Squeeze real hard, 1-2-3-4-5. Now let the lemon drop to the floor. Relax your hand, 1-2-3-4-5. One more time, squeeze real hard, 1-2-3-4-5. Now let the lemon drop to the floor. Relax your hand, 1-2-3-4-5. Squeeze again, 1-2-3-4-5, and let go, 1-2-3-4-5.

Next, take your left hand and squeeze the lemon. That's it, try to get all the juice out of the lemon, 1-2-3-4-5.

Now, let the lemon drop. Relax your hand. Feel your hand relax. Squeeze again, 1-2-3-4-5, and let go, 1-2-3-4-5. One more time, squeeze real hard, 1-2-3-4-5. Now let the lemon drop to the floor, and relax.

Good. You may be starting to feel relaxed already.

3. Shoulders:

Now I want you to try to make your shoulders touch your ears. Squeeze your head into your shoulders, like a turtle going into its shell. That's it. Now relax your shoulders. Drop them down as low as they can go. One more time, try to make your shoulders touch your ears, hold it, 1-2-3-4-5, good. Now relax your shoulders, 1-2-3-4-5.

4. Neck:

Turn your head all the way to the left. Good, now slowly turn your head all the way to the right. Now put your head down so that your chin is touching your chest, and now put your head all the way back. Good. Now let your arms hang down and shake them and loosen your shoulders.

5. Arms:

Now take your arms and reach for the ceiling, try to touch the ceiling. Hold your hands up real high, as high as you can go, 1-2-3-4-5.

Good. Now let your arms drop to your sides, 1-2-3-4-5. Give 'em a little shake if you'd like.

Now reach up to the ceiling again, *reach*, as high as you can. Good. Now drop your arms to your sides.

6. Stomach:

Next I want you to squeeze in your tummy, like you're doing a sit-up or trying to squeeze through a narrow slot in a fence, make your tummy really flat and tight, 1-2-3-4-5.

Good, now relax your tummy, 1-2-3-4-5. Okay, squeeze it one more time, make it really tight, 1-2-3-4-5. Good! And relax.

7. Legs:

Now I want you to take your right thigh and squeeze really tight, 1-2-3-4-5.

Good. Now relax and count to five, 1-2-3-4-5. Squeeze again, hold it. Good. Relax.

Now squeeze your left thigh. Squeeze really hard, 1-2-3-4-5. Now relax, 1-2-3-4-5. Squeeze again, hold it. Good. Relax.

8. Feet:

Next—your feet and toes. Try to curl your toes down as far as you can, like you're digging them into squishy mud. Hold them there, 1-2-3-4-5. Good. Now relax your toes, 1-2-3-4-5. Now curl them down again, as far as you can.

If you're having trouble curling your toes, you can put your feet on the floor and push your feet and toes into the floor as hard as you can. Good. Relax your toes.

In a few seconds we'll be finished. You did a *great* job. Did you notice the difference between when you were tight and when you were relaxed?

This script was designed for kids ages seven through thirteen, but as we mentioned earlier, you should use the language that you feel suits your child best. Progressive muscle relaxation and diaphragmatic breathing techniques benefit all ages. You can also add other muscles in the body, like the buttocks and calves. See how long your child is able to stay focused on this practice; you can decide whether to add more.

There are more relaxation exercises, as well as kids showing how to do the exercises, in our computer program, *Camp Cope-A-Lot* at CopingCatParents.com. This activity was designed to help youth reduce anxiety. The program includes scenes that walk a child through progressive muscle relaxation and diaphragmatic breathing. You can learn to relax by watching this, and then use what you've learned to teach your child. Or you can show it to your child and let them watch and learn on their own. You can also download the audio (mp3) so your child can follow along on their own.

Technique 3: Guided Imagery

Imagery can also be very helpful, especially when combined with the physical relaxation methods like diaphragmatic breathing. To reduce stress with imagery, you use your imagination to recreate and enjoy a very relaxing situation. The more intensely you imagine the situation, the more relaxing the experience will be.

One common use of guided imagery is to imagine a scene, place, or event that you remember as safe, peaceful, restful, beautiful, and happy. You can bring all your senses into the imagery with, for example, sounds of running water and birds, the smell of cut grass, the taste of cool lemonade, the warmth of the sun, and so on. Use the imagined place as a retreat from stress and pressure. Collaborating with your child, you can gently and patiently talk about calming places. You may have your opinions, but let your child choose their own calming image. It's less critical that you agree that it is a calming image, and more important that your child thinks of it as a calming image. One of our young patients chose an amusement park for their calm place. Although we may not consider this calming, the child identified it as a place they felt relaxed and happy. It actually worked out great because there were many beautiful sounds and scenes that could be described.

Scenes can involve a complex setting such as an ocean beach. You may see cliffs, the ocean and sand around you, hear the waves crashing against rocks, smell the salt in the air, and feel the warmth of the sun and a gentle breeze on your body. Other images might include imagining blowing up a balloon, letting it go and watching it fly into the sky and float away, then filling up another balloon, and another, until the sky fills up with different colored balloons.

Here is an example of how you can lead your child through guided imagery. You are the primary speaker; your child is meant to use your words as prompts to guide their imagining.

1. What do you see? See the sun in the sky, and you're surrounded by blue skies. There's no one else around. The leaves are glistening in the trees.

2. What do you hear? You can hear the birds chirping and the leaves rustling as the breeze flows through them.

3. What do you feel? You can feel the warm sun on your face. Your hair gently falls across your forehead. The breeze feels slightly cool on your skin.

4. What do you smell? You can smell the fresh air, the fresh-cut grass, and the fragrance of nearby flowers.

5. What do you taste? You have a glass of iced lemonade that's sweet and tart and makes your mouth tingle.

Other relaxing imagery may involve creating mental pictures of stress flowing out of your body. For example, you can imagine the color blue washing over you and carrying all of your stress away.

A Few Things to Keep in Mind

You can teach your child how to relax using these scripts, or you can rely more on the videos in *Camp Cope-A-Lot*. Neither method is better than the other—it's your call. Either way, the goal is for your child to learn the skills to be better able to relax. As your child learns how to relax, they will become more aware of their muscle tension and other physical sensations of stress and anxiety. Once your child knows what stress feels like, they can make a conscious effort to practice relaxation the moment they start to feel stress. This approach can prevent stress from spiraling into more severe anxiety and distress.

Remember that relaxation is a skill—and as with any skill, the ability to relax improves with practice. Keep in mind that relaxation is best practiced, at least initially, in a nonstressful situation. Once some skill has been mastered, relaxation can be a strategy to practice when your child wants to reduce overall stress and physical tension. It usually works best to make it part of their normal routine. For example, if your child is on a sports team, they can practice relaxation as part of their cooldown routine after practice. Or if they have a bedtime routine of getting into pajamas and reading, relaxation practice can become part of it. As with all the steps of the FEAR plan, we recommend finishing off the practice session with an activity of your child's choosing (yes, even if they choose video games!). That way they'll associate this time with a positive experience, reinforcing the effort.

That said, it's important to not send the message to use relaxation strategies to "escape" anxiety or as a quick fix to try to make the bad feelings go away. Remember, we don't want your child to try to prevent all anxiety or seek immediate relief from anxiety. Rather, we want them to learn that when they feel anxious or stressed, they have ways to cope. It's true that these techniques serve to immediately calm heightened arousal, but if we try to use the strategies as a quick fix to make panic or arousal go away, rather than for preparing to approach or challenge our worries, we could be inadvertently sending our brains the message that we are in danger. Relaxation is a strategy to practice so that your child can reduce overall stress and physical tension—not a strategy to *control* these physical symptoms. So rather than saying, "You're panicking and you need to calm down. Why don't you do your relaxation practice?" you can remind them that "It's okay to take a couple of deep belly breaths if you're feeling anxious—it will help to refocus on the present and begin to challenge the worry and decide what you want to do next." Again, we don't want to use relaxation to try to stop all anxiety or to seek immediate relief from anxiety.

Again, you're not a lecturing teacher, but a guiding coach. Be patient—don't let failure, a setback, or refusal to practice relaxation become yet another stressor. It can be extremely difficult to focus on just one thing—our minds naturally wander (even as adults), and it's understandable that a young child can become agitated or bored when they're being asked to sit still in one place but their mind and their body's inclinations are straying elsewhere.

Don't pressure your child or feel you need to remind them to practice every day. As long as you've shared the skills, practiced with them a few times, and helped them make it part of their routine, your job is done—you've provided guidance, support, and encouragement. When you make these helpful practices a demand, it takes away from your child's internal motivation to practice. Without that, sooner or later they will drop the practice anyway. As long as they know how to use the tool, they will know they have something in their toolkit that they can use, and with time they'll learn the connection between the skill and reduced anxiety. That will be the true motivator for practice in the long term.

Keep in mind, there are lots of situations where some tension is normal and to be expected. You're at a sporting event, and your team is behind by only a small bit, and you are in a position to improve your team's score. You're about to go on stage to deliver your lines. Our kids can't avoid all stress, nor would we want them to. We are helping them develop skills to manage it. These relaxation strategies are a great life skill for training our bodies to stay out of unwarranted fight-or-flight mode as much as possible.

For Kids with More Chronic Anxiety

One feature of distressing and maladaptive anxiety is that the person brings a tense style to everyday nonstressful activities, and sometimes even to the activities that should be relaxing. When a child is persistently anxious, their sympathetic nervous system may always be poised to react to a crisis, putting them in a state of persistent tension. They will be vulnerable to reacting to small stresses the same way they would reasonably react to real emergencies. Repeated episodes of the fight-or-flight reaction that comes with anxiety can deplete energy and, if they continue, can be exhausting.

As we mentioned earlier, many children who live with high levels of anxiety breathe shallowly, only in their chest. Shallow breathing with the chest can lead to an imbalance of oxygen and carbon dioxide in the system and can initiate or maintain a physical sense of anxiety. Shallow, quick breaths cause physical responses such as increased heart rate and blood pressure. For these kids, progressive muscle relaxation and breathing retraining are particularly helpful.

Meditation

Many people ask us about the difference between relaxation training, meditation, and mindfulness. There are many similarities and the practices do overlap, but the terms are not interchangeable.

It's easy to see why the terms are often confused. They all involve the practice of focusing attention to achieve increased self-awareness, and they all have a secondary benefit of calming the mind and body and have positive effects including improved mood and resilience and better sleep. The difference lies in their intention as well as in how they are practiced. When deciding which technique to practice and when, it's important to be clear about the intention of the practice.

The intention of relaxation training is to develop the skill of creating physiological calm and reducing overall arousal. In contrast, the ancient practice of meditation is intended to develop the skill of focus, to cultivate awareness and calm or transcend mind chatter. This skill can help in many ways, but the goal of meditation is to build and practice the skill itself. This focus could be on anything—on a single object, a sound, or nothingness. The focus could also be on your breath—which is why it sometimes becomes difficult to tease meditation apart from deep breathing or belly breathing practice. Seated meditation usually begins with deep breathing in a comfortable position, and you can spend a minute to an hour or more in which you practice focus. With regular use, meditation helps you become more aware of both your thoughts and the meanings you assign to things, and your body, ultimately giving you more clarity and stability. Meditation can also be practiced in movement—yoga is one example. The different forms of meditation practice all have this in common: they give the mind something simple on which to focus, to train and condition the mind to observe with calm and clarity—to go above and beyond our normal mental processes.

Guided Meditation

Here is an example of a guided meditation technique that works well for kids:

Have you ever noticed that when you're quiet, that your mind is not really quiet? That it is really going and thinking about a lot of things? Your mind is like a little puppy—it wants to run all over the place, but it is possible to bring your puppy back close to you and have it go where you ask. Let's practice training your mind to stay on the path with you. We're going to practice paying attention to one thing—we'll start by practicing to pay attention to your breath.

1. Sit down comfortably and close your eyes.

2. Bring all of your attention to your breath and slow it down, take a deep breath, and then slowly exhale through your nose.

3. Ask your mind to follow the breath. Every time your mind wanders away, lead it back to the sound and feeling of your breathing. Follow your breath as you inhale and exhale.

4. Count each breath at the end of every exhale. We're going to go up to 10.

5. Don't let your mind count before the end of the exhale. The puppy always wants to jump ahead, but don't let it. Bring it back on the path and follow your breath.

When you've reached the end and counted to 10, stay still and spend a few minutes in quiet, encouraging your child to keep breathing slow and steady.

Mindfulness

Dr. Jon Kabat-Zinn has studied and brought attention to the practice of mindfulness for reduction of stress. The term *mindfulness*, for awareness, comes from the same traditions as the practice of meditation. Kabat-Zinn has defined mindfulness as "the awareness that arises through paying attention, on purpose, in the present moment, nonjudgmentally." The intention of mindfulness is to practice awareness of what is going on in and around you in the present moment and nonjudgmentally observing it. When you are being actively mindful, you are noticing and paying attention to your thoughts, feelings, behaviors, and movements, and also to the effect you have on those around you. Living mindfully means that you are a more aware participant in every moment and more compassionate and accepting of your inner and outer world.

You can practice mindfulness anytime, anywhere, and with anyone by being fully engaged in the here and now. When most people go about their daily lives, their minds wander from the actual activity they are participating in to other thoughts or sensations. When you're mindful, you are actively involved in the activity with all of your senses instead of allowing your mind to wander.

Things get confusing when there is mention of *mindfulness meditation*. But by now you can see that mindfulness can be done in the form of meditation, and meditation involves being mindful, but mindfulness does not require meditation, and meditation as a skill aims to focus beyond the present moment. Mindfulness can be practiced both informally (at any time/place) and formally (during meditation). Whereas meditation is usually practiced for a specific amount of time, mindfulness can be applied to any situation throughout the day. Mindfulness meditation uses meditation techniques, such as focus on your breath or an object, to practice nonjudgmental awareness of the present—everything you are thinking, seeing, feeling, and hearing in the moment. Mindfulness-based stress reduction (MBSR), developed by Kabat-Zinn in the 1970s, is a formalized eight-week course on using mindfulness to reduce stress. The following is an example of a mindfulness practice you can teach your child.

Mindful Eating

You like chocolate, right? When is the last time you really, truly enjoyed a piece of chocolate? We usually eat quickly, enjoy the sweetness, and then forget all about it. We miss out on so much of the real joy and pleasure of it. It's like we're missing out on how great chocolate really is! Let's see if we can try to really enjoy chocolate by using all of our senses—sight, hearing, touch, smell, and taste. For each sense, name two or three things you notice about the chocolate.

1. Give a piece of chocolate to your child, and you have one as well to guide the focus.

2. Okay, lets look at it: what do you see? (Yes, I see that too. I also noticed my fingers are getting chocolate on them as the chocolate is slowly melting.)

3. Let's put it in our mouths now. Describe the flavor of the chocolate on your tongue.

4. Can you describe anything about the smell of the chocolate? (I can smell the aroma of coming through my nostrils.)

5. What do you notice about how it feels? (It's really gooey and smooth in my mouth.)

6. Do you notice anything about your tongue? (I can feel my tongue tingle as it tastes the chocolate, and I can feel saliva forming.)

7. Did you feel like closing your eyes too? (It's almost like my mind wanted to focus so much on the taste, it didn't want to be disturbed by what's happening on the outside.)

8. What do you hear? What sounds does it makes when you're chewing? (Chewy, slurpy.)

A similar exercise is the mindfulness walk. You can walk around your backyard or along a trail and practice noticing things using all five senses. These practices are intended to help your child tune in to their surroundings and increase their present-moment awareness. As with all of the techniques we've discussed, it's important that you are patient and keep it fun and peaceful. If they are taking a long time to focus, that's okay. It's normal to get off track; then you'll work to guide them back to noticing, slowly and gently, and with a smile.

Is Exercise Enough?

Many parents ask, if their child is already involved in sports or dance or a physical activity that increases blood flow and improves breathing and sends signals to their brain that they are safe and happy, is this sufficient? Can exercise replace the need to do separate breathing or relaxation practices for the purposes of reducing stress and cutting off stress response?

Exercise is certainly important and beneficial for anxiety management, focus, resilience, and overall well-being, but the intention of each of these techniques is more than cutting off the stress response and increasing feel-good endorphins. They help to improve our control over our mind processes. They also show the important connection between our focus and our physiology and emotional experience. Control over our focus is very much a key skill of resilience.

Relaxation training, meditation, and mindfulness techniques address only part of what maintains stress and anxiety. They are necessary but not sufficient by themselves in helping our kids manage stress and challenges throughout their lives. If we think again about the things that contribute to anxiety and negative mood, these include beliefs, interpretations, and behaviors. Without also adding awareness and control over beliefs and behaviors, it's unlikely that minimizing fight-or-flight response will be effective over the long term. It's important to gain insight and to modify patterns of behaviors that maintain anxiety and low mood.

Key Takeaways

We don't want to need to go to a beach to feel relaxed. Planning an escape sends our body the message that we are not okay—that it's time to "flee." We want to feel relaxed before going to the beach.

Benefits of Relaxation:

- Slowing your heart rate

- Lowering blood pressure

- Slowing your breathing rate

- Increasing blood flow to major muscles

- Reducing muscle tension and pain

- Improving concentration

- Improving sleep

- Boosting confidence to handle problems

Doing a form of relaxation every day for a few weeks helps build up our reserves to stay in a more relaxed state and makes it even easier and faster to send the *everything is okay* message to our brain.

Relaxation training, meditation, and mindfulness have many similarities and overlaps, but the terms are not interchangeable.

- Relaxation training develops the skill of creating physiological calm and reducing overall arousal.

- Meditation is an ancient practice intended to develop the skill of focus in order to cultivate awareness and transcend mind chatter.

- Mindfulness—"the awareness that arises through paying attention, on purpose, in the present moment, nonjudgmentally"—can take the form of meditation, and meditation involves being mindful, but mindfulness does not require meditation, and meditation aims to focus beyond the present moment.

All three techniques are necessary but not sufficient to help our kids manage stress and challenges throughout their lives. It's important to gain insight and to modify patterns of behaviors that maintain anxiety and low mood.

CHAPTER 7

The E Step: Expecting Bad Things to Happen?

The greatest discovery of any generation is that a human can alter his life by altering his attitude.

—William James

When we assume that the world is acting on us and we are just living in response, we lose the opportunity to create our experience. We find ourselves in struggle, just trying to stay above water, going moment by moment, experiencing emotions and helpless in terms of what happens next. "My job is not fulfilling, and the job market is terrible" or "My [spouse/partner] just doesn't give me what I need from them," or "My kids aren't trying hard enough in school." Being focused on day-to-day struggles and anticipating future struggle is how we maintain stress and drain ourselves emotionally and physically. But if we keep in mind that whatever we are feeling is coming from our thoughts—from where we've put our focus, from our interpretation of events, and based on beliefs that have been built over years, not necessarily the "truth"—it means we can change it. There's not just one way to see things, and therefore not just one way to feel.

Using Our Superpower

As part of your own journey as your child's coach, keep in mind, as often as you can, that in each situation, it is your thoughts that create your emotional experience, your "reality"—not the situation or the outside world. Your thoughts in the moment *seem* to be just what is. They seem true, they seem to be a mirror for what is happening—of your reality. But think of the CBT model introduced in chapter 1: your thoughts are coming from a well of your previous experiences and beliefs—your stories—as much as they are coming from the moment. There are no "truths." There are just many interpretations.

You may recall that individuals have not all had the same response to the COVID-19 pandemic, not only because of individual differences in our circumstances, but because our thoughts, or how we interpreted the situation, were different.

Situation	Thought	Feeling
Lockdown	*I can't do all the things that I love to do or see the people that make my life fun.* *What if I get sick? How would I protect the kids? What if I'm among those who have a fatal reaction?*	Depressed Anxious

> *I wake up with a headache; I feel defeated already.*
>
> *I have a meeting with my boss later in the day, so I feel anxious.*
>
> *I'm living in lockdown and can't guarantee my well-being or the well-being of those I love, so I feel depressed, scared, and trapped.*

While we don't have the power to control others, or the world around us, we do have the power to control the direction and focus of our thoughts and, from there, our subsequent actions. Which means that we have the power to create our experience. Remember, we have a superpower. Our mind's ability to think—to create, plan, imagine, see things with our imagination that we have never seen and even those that have never existed, is our greatest strength. It allows for innovation and limitless progress. It allows us to learn from past mistakes and improve future outcomes. It also allows us to choose our focus and choose our response.

Situation	Thought	Feeling
Lockdown	*I'm so grateful to wake up healthy.*	Grateful
	I have a chance to spend some time playing outside with my kids.	Hopeful
	I will do what I need to do to take care of myself and my family.	

You can *choose* to take a wider view—a big-picture perspective. Only then will you be in position to be focused on a goal. We often think that we will be able to focus on our goals only after we have eliminated all the problems standing in our way, but that's where we can get stuck in a worry cycle. For example, you are planning a family vacation. As you start thinking of dates and hotels, you also begin thinking of other potential problems—weather, illness, getting lost, problems with your room, and so on. You can spend two full weeks before your trip thinking of potential problems and trying to think of solutions. You are thinking that if you can eliminate 99 percent of the problems before your trip, you'll enjoy the vacation more. Your energy and focus are on the problems that may arise. This starts your worry cycle—the alarm goes off, you try to solve the problem (*I'll call the hotel tomorrow to make sure the room has what we need*), and you feel a bit better. But then your body learns that you are in danger and starts scanning for more danger, and more and more potential problems come to mind, and more and more alarms go off. When you get there, the chances are you'll already be stressed and tired, and there will still inevitably be problems that pop up. You will have less energy and patience to handle these otherwise manageable problems. Your reality will be that this was a stressful vacation—not a vacation at all.

Instead, focusing on the goal and knowing that you'll handle things as they come, rather than anticipating and preventing them, may be the fastest and easiest path to creating more of what you want. This approach also serves to teach your body that you are not in danger—keeping you feeling calm and confident longer with fewer false alarms. In this case, the goal is to enjoy some down time with your family and create some new memories. Focusing on that, and knowing that you are in the driver's seat of creating it, takes you out of the worry cycle. *The weather may be bad, but we'll make the best of it. We might get lost, but we'll figure it out. As long as we're all together, we'll be making memories. We're so lucky to have the opportunity to travel.*

Push yourself to practice choosing your response before approaching different situations, and see what experiences you can create. For example, you can plan a phone call to your parent or older relative to say hello and check in. Before you make the call, choose the emotion you'd like to create (say, joy) and then choose to focus on the aspect of your relationship that brings you joy (say, gratitude for the many sacrifices they've made). Choose to give your love unconditionally. Keep in perspective the factors that go into the situation (they may criticize, but that is an old habit to "parent" you, and that's how they show their love. You know who you are; you don't need to adjust their opinion of who you are). When you make the call, remember to choose to focus on gratitude, instead of giving in to your first automatic reaction to the situation (for example, if they criticize you, stay focused on their years of sacrifice; it's just their way of showing love, so you proceed with creating joy, instead of getting angry or seeking an apology). You can practice and become a model of believing in the power of choice in creating the life you want, rather than taking an approach of reacting to events as they come.

The fact that it doesn't seem automatic—that you may have to force yourself, or struggle with staying with that focus—isn't a sign that you are not genuine or that it's not true. The struggle is normal. Our initial automatic responses have formed over many years, and habits of thinking have formed. In times when we are anxious, remember that it is more our "bully" telling us to watch out, to reflect on past mistakes, and less that we are in imminent danger. It's normal that we have to fight back—but it's a battle worth fighting to remind ourselves that we are okay; we are not in immediate harm, and if need be, we can problem solve. But we'll do that only if we are faced with a genuine problem, not in anticipation of the problem.

Kids are more vulnerable to quickly giving in to the idea that we are just responding to the world rather than in control of our response than adults are, because of their level of cognitive development and their more limited life experience. They are in the developmental stage of moving from concrete thinking to more abstract thinking but are still very black and white—seeing things as good or bad, right or wrong, in their control or out of their control—when interpreting events and choosing their response. They also do not have as much ability to think long term; they're not usually thinking about what their response would mean for their future or how it's impacting their own growth and character development.

But they still have the same superpower: the ability to choose their response. We want to give them the gift of awareness of this power—to show them how much they are in control of their moment.

We also want to offer them a way to get "unstuck" from worry and rumination—the thought processes that lead to anxiety and depression. Remember, our ability to think is also our kryptonite—our complex and imaginative minds allow us to linger longer on our mistakes, our disappointments, our weaknesses. We can feel anxious and miserable any time we choose to focus on what we *don't* have, what we *can't* do, how things will never change, and how we have been wronged.

We will share with them that we don't have to just react to situations, we can challenge our initial "automatic" response—"It might be a false alarm!" or "Watch out! The bully is trying to get your attention!"—and choose our response. We don't have to just react to situations; we can choose our perspective. We can choose our focus—choose to focus on what we *do* have, and what we *can* do, rather than what we are lacking. We can choose to not give up. We can choose to be resilient.

Thinking About Thinking

One of the main benefits of talk therapy is the opportunity it provides to think about our thinking and to receive support in generating and considering alternative perspectives and choosing our response. In this chapter, we are recommending that you create opportunities to talk, think about thoughts, and consider alternative perspectives with your child at home.

The E step helps your child notice their thoughts or self-talk so that they can build self-awareness and be in a position to evaluate and choose their response. It also reminds them that the bully might be scanning for danger and that they may be **E**xpecting bad things to happen more often than expecting good things to happen—which throws off their focus and control over their experience. They can use the E step to regain that control.

CONVERSATION STARTER   The last couple of weeks we've been talking a lot about feelings and trying to understand how and why our body feels the way it does when we are sad or nervous. You are getting to be a real expert in naming and understanding feelings. We are now good at the first step of the FEAR plan, the F step—asking ourselves "What am I **F**eeling?" With the next step of the FEAR plan, the E step, we're going to become experts when it comes to understanding thoughts. How are thoughts different from feelings? Some say feelings come from our heart and thoughts come from our mind.

You may not notice it, but in your mind, you are saying things to yourself all the time. These are our thoughts, the things we say to ourselves without speaking out loud. Some people call it our *inner voice*, others call it our *self-talk*. In our mind we are having thoughts about what we've learned, what we've decided, what we are planning, what we remember, what we think about different situations...all the time. But we don't usually stop to think about our thinking.

Your Thoughts Affect How You Feel

From here, you can introduce the idea that it's not just the situation that makes us feel how we feel, but our interpretation, or how we think about the situation, that makes us feel that way. You can start with an experiment to show them how powerful their thoughts are.

CONVERSATION STARTER   It's really important to notice what you are thinking, because what you are thinking—the things that you are picturing, or your inner voice—is really powerful in affecting how you feel. Whenever you are having a feeling, there's probably a thought that goes with it.

Let's do a little experiment. Let's try to listen to our self-talk for a minute. Sometimes it will be images, other times it might be that we can hear the words we are saying to ourselves.

Now imagine for a minute that this was the last day of school and your teacher just announced that it was time to pack up. How do you feel? What are you picturing? Did you notice that just by thinking about something, you created a feeling in just a few seconds? What thoughts do you hear in your mind? If it's hard to know exactly what you were thinking, think of how you feel and then ask yourself, *what was I just thinking about or picturing that made me feel this way?*

Then give an example of a situation where different people are feeling differently—even though they are in the same situation. This serves as proof that the situation isn't the only thing involved in how we feel; it's also how we're thinking about the situation. You can give a real-life example that you and your child might remember, or just a general example like this one:

It's easy to think that our feelings come from whatever situation we are in. You might assume, if you're at a birthday party with friends, that because you're in that situation you'll feel happy. But it's really how you're thinking about the situation (your self-talk) that makes you feel the way you feel— no matter the situation. Take the birthday party as an example—can you imagine that not everyone at the party is feeling happy? Even though they are all at a party, everyone is feeling something different. It might be that someone is feeling nervous because they don't know any of the other kids and are not sure how to make friends. Someone else might be bored because they don't like the kinds of activities at the party. Someone else might be sad because they didn't get picked to be on the team they wanted when the kids were playing games. These kids all feel differently, but not because they are in a different situation—it's because they are all thinking about different things. They feel differently based on what they are focused on. *It's not just the situation that makes us feel a certain way; it's what we are thinking about the situation that makes us feel that way.*

The E Step: Expecting Bad Things to Happen?

Most worry, stress, and bad feelings come from thoughts anticipating unwanted outcomes or future "bad" things, and from reflecting on expectations that weren't met. Disappointment happens primarily when we are set on a specific expectation. This is why social comparison is so damaging. We use the example of another person's experience to set expectations for ourselves. We then interpret and experience anything other than the expected outcome as a failure. Fear comes from an expectation of a future unwanted event.

Instead of going with your child's initial "automatic" expectation of a bad thing happening (or focusing on a bad thing that happened), we hope that they challenge that thought—making sure it's consistent with what they really think, it's putting things in perspective, it's accurate, and most important, it's useful.

The E step in the FEAR plan stands for "Expecting bad things to happen?" In the E step, we are reminding children to think about what they are thinking, remembering that that thought is part of the reason they feel how they feel, and that it is time to check whether or not that thought is the most accurate and most helpful thought to have in that moment.

CONVERSATION STARTER When we're feeling worried, we are quick to assume that it's the situation that makes us worry—like it's the book report that is due, or it's because there's a big game coming up. You may think that it's the situation that makes you feel a certain way, but it's really how you are thinking about the situation (your self-talk) that makes you feel the way you feel.

Need some convincing? Well, imagine that two kids are both in class when the teacher announces, "Surprise! We're going to an amusement park for a field trip next week!"

Situation	Thought	Feeling
We're going to an amusement park!	*I hate roller coasters. Everyone will go and give me a hard time. I'll be the only one just waiting on the bench all day. I don't want to go!*	Worried/Sad
We're going to an amusement park!	*I love roller coasters! I can't wait to have cotton candy and a day of hanging out with friends!*	Excited/Happy

Though they are both in the same situation, the students have different thoughts about the teacher's surprise, and therefore they feel very differently.

It's our thoughts about the situation that cause our bodies to go into fight-or-flight mode. We want things to go smoothly, so as soon as we think *what if it doesn't?*, our body's alarm goes off and we feel stressed or worried.

Just the way our body alarm goes off and gets us ready to run, our minds get ready for danger too. We start to think about all the bad things that could happen. Have you noticed, when you're worried or sad, you're thinking about all the bad things that could happen in your day, or all the things you don't want? Like, *That test is going to be really hard*, or *If I don't score, the team is going to think I can't play*, or *What if my mom forgets to pick me up?* (Use an example here that would be relevant and familiar to your child.)

As soon as you notice that you are **F**eeling anxious, sad, or any big feeling, it's time to go to the E step of the FEAR plan. The E step is when you to ask yourself: *Am I **E**xpecting bad things to happen?* If the answer is yes, you are *thinking* about bad things that could happen or did happen. *Keep in mind: just because you thought it, doesn't mean you think it!* It might be a false alarm.

Give your child some tips to identify worries and negative thoughts: Worries often start with the words "What if..."

What if I mess up and everyone makes fun of me?

What if I get sick in school? What if I throw up?

What if I miss my parents and I want to come home?

What if I get a bad grade and my parents get angry with me?

Sad thoughts are usually about not being good enough, or that things will never change, or that things will always be bad. They usually include the words *can't, everything, never,* or *always...*

I can't run as fast as the other kids.

I'm not good at talking to people.

I'm so bored with everything.

I never get invited to anything.

I always do worse than all the other kids.

Your goal is to build their awareness of their pattern or style of thinking. We know that even our own thinking becomes habit over time. Help your child become more aware of their habits or patterns of thinking by helping them come up with a list of their most common worries or sad thoughts. We sometimes call these *frequent fliers* because they fly through our minds often—more out of habit than out of an active process of thinking.

Let's list some of the *What if, I can't, I never, I always,* or *I should* thoughts that you notice most often in your self-talk (or let's write these down in your journal). It's good for us to know the frequent flier thoughts that pop up for you, because then you'll be able to handle them more quickly the next time they come up.

Challenging Negative or Anxious Thoughts

It's a great skill to be able to step back from your initial response and look at it, judge it, and decide what you want to do with it. This skill helps us put things in perspective, problem solve, and move forward. As you're discussing these "what if" and "always" thoughts, it's also important to normalize this experience—to explain that everyone has these thoughts flying in from time to time, and we all have to challenge them so they don't stop us from doing what we need to do.

CONVERSATION STARTER   It can seem as if worries help us prepare or plan to make sure nothing bad happens or to find a way to fix things that did happen. But when you're "**E**xpecting something bad to happen" or thinking about something bad that happened, you're usually just taking time away from what you really need or want to do. These are unhelpful thoughts that won't help you solve your problem and won't help you feel better.

I want to give you a list of some frequent flier thoughts that all of us have. This way you'll be quick to challenge them rather than letting them stick around and stop you from doing what you want to do.

Common warning messages your false alarm might be sending:

- **Don't go!** Stay away from situations that could be uncomfortable. It's going to be scary. You won't have fun. There could be mean adults or mean kids there. You might need something and no one will be able to help. You might feel sick and you won't be able to handle it.

- **You have the worst luck.** It's going to be the worst! Always thinking the *worst ever* is going to happen. You'll fail the test.

You'll mess up, and everyone will laugh, and you'll never be able to live it down. It's the most important test of your whole life, and it will ruin your entire future. No one likes you.

- **It will always be bad.** Remember last time? It happened once, so it's always going to happen that way. You'll never improve. This will never get easier. No one will ever like you.

- **You're not good enough!** You aren't smart enough, funny enough, good looking enough. Everyone else can do it, except you. Everyone is doing things easily, except you.

- **The shoulds.** You really *should* do everything better! You *should* have worked harder. You *should* be more confident. You *should* be more outgoing. You *shouldn't* make mistakes. All of your essays and projects *should* be the best.

- **Mistakes are *not* okay!** If you get a bad grade, everyone will think you're stupid. If you forget your homework, you'll get in trouble. If you don't do it right, everyone will be disappointed.

- **No one really likes you.** You never say or do the right thing. People don't like you; they think you're weird. Everyone has friends except you. If you try to say something, they'll think you're lame. Everyone is thinking and saying mean things about you behind your back.

Why is your brain so mean sometimes? It thinks it's protecting you from bad things by saying these things—but actually it just makes you feel sad and worried. It's time to ignore the false alarm!

Instead of listening to the thoughts about what bad things might happen or how something didn't go the way you had hoped, you can challenge your worries so they won't take time away from focusing on doing what you want or need to be doing.

Practice using these "challenge" questions whenever your alarm is going off or when one of your worries is popping up and interrupting your day (or night):

- What are all the things that could happen? The good things? Bad things?

- I've had this worry before—what usually happens?

- Just because I think it doesn't mean it's true. Is this thought the most accurate or the most useful thought I could have in this situation?

- My worry thought always says that if this goes badly, my life will be ruined. But is this really a life-ruining situation? Or just a tough situation?

- Worry likes to use old tricks to get me to pay attention. Is this a false alarm?

- Do I have to pay attention to this thought? What was I doing before this worry popped up?

- Is this useful to be thinking about right now? How much time do I want to spend thinking about it in this way?

- I can't control what ends up happening, but I can control what I choose to think, feel, and do. What do I want to do about this?

- Things might go really well. I'm pretty good at this, and I've already achieved success in many ways.

Here's an example:

Self-Talk: Today was a terrible day. Am I really happy with my life?

- By asking this question, you are focused on being not happy, which keeps you feeling unhappy.

- More helpful and accurate: All days have good parts, bad parts, boring parts, sad parts, happy parts, whatever parts. Which part do you want to spend more time on?

Self-Talk: School is *hard*; I don't have time for myself, I don't have time for anything I enjoy!

- School is hard sometimes, but pursuing our goals is a great source of fulfillment.

- More helpful and accurate: It is hard, but I wouldn't choose something day after day that was *not* challenging me.

Choose Your Focus

It's important to remember that you control the focus of your thoughts. You decide what your mind zooms in on, and that's how you can choose how you want to feel.

How you feel comes from your attitude, or how you're thinking about things. So if you choose to think about all the good things in your life, the people you love, the things you enjoy doing, or the good things in a situation, you'll feel good. When we focus on what we don't have, what we can't do, what didn't go well, or what might turn out badly, we tend to feel sad and worried. When focusing on what happened in the past, our brains tend to magnify the bad things and minimize the good things. We are more likely to remember something not so great rather than something really great. If you focus on something bad that could happen in the future, or the bad things about a situation, you'll feel worried, nervous, anxious, or sad. On the other hand, if you focus on something you feel lucky to have or on something good that lies ahead, you'll feel calm, happy, or even excited. We aren't saying you should think everything is great all the time. However, we want your thoughts to be accurate—not overpredicting or focusing on bad possibilities.

CONVERSATION STARTER   In the moment it seems like whatever thought pops up is just true. Like that's just the situation we're in, and that's all there is to it. But there are a million things that are also true in every situation and maybe even more true. Remember, just because you thought it, doesn't mean you think it! Like, if you ever had the thought *I never get invited to anything*, your thought is focused on a few specific events—times that you were not invited to something you wanted to go to. But that thought is leaving out all of the invitations you have had and will have. It's leaving out that invitations change with different times in the year, changes in other people's lives, changes in schools or friend groups, and changes as you get older. That thought is leaving out that invitations are not the way to measure that you are loved. It's forgetting all the people in the world who love you. It's leaving out that you can be an inviter if you ever want to have something fun planned with a friend.

This scenario gives an example of invitation, but you can use a thought that is a frequent flier for your child and use that as the starting point to show what their initial, automatic thought is leaving out.

In every situation, we can say unhelpful things to ourselves: thoughts that make us feel unsure, sad, and afraid—or we can say helpful things to ourselves that make us feel confident, calm, and ready. We want to be good at reminding ourselves of the things that are true—the things that help us stay confident, calm, and ready—as often and as quickly as possible. We always want our self-talk to be as accurate and useful as it can be. After we challenge our anxious thoughts, come up with more accurate and useful thoughts to help you feel less worried throughout the day.

Hints for finding the most useful and accurate thoughts:

- *This is temporary.* Will I be thinking about this when I'm older? Every day brings some good things and some bad things. This won't matter for long; the people I love are what really matter. There are so many good things ahead.

- *I can't fail, because I'll never stop trying.* There are no losses or wrong choices; I can only learn from my experiences and keep getting better.

- *Think about all the things in a situation, not just the "bad" parts.* I may not have won the race, but I beat my time from last week. By improving a skill each week, I'll have a better chance of winning more races later.

- *It's not usually black/white—it's more gray.* For instance, I'm not usually going to fail; I might get a few things wrong. Or I'm usually not going to need to go to the hospital, but I might need some medicine and rest for a few days.

- *We're human; we can't expect to never mess up.* I'm going to forget, misunderstand, make mistakes. I can't expect to do everything perfectly. I've handled it before when things don't go perfectly.

- *These are not my chosen thoughts and feelings.* So I will choose to not pay attention to them. I can wait this out and not give time and attention to the thoughts that are coming from worry.

- *I am in full control of my actions.* Worry and sadness are emotions; they cannot make me do anything or stop me from doing anything. I will continue to do the things, even if it's uncomfortable or challenging.

- *If someone says or thinks something negative about me or to me, that is their problem.* They are bringing negativity into their world. I don't need to feed their negativity. I will stay focused on the people and things that bring positivity to my world.

When you worry, you start focusing on all the things you can't do and all the things you don't have. Don't let your worries bully you. Instead, try to focus your thoughts on the things you can do and all the things you do have. Practice thinking of more accurate and useful thoughts. Use the Challenging Worry Worksheet (available for download at http://www. newharbinger.com/46967) to identify a worry, challenge it, and find a more useful and accurate thought.

If we fill our thoughts with what we don't have and what we don't want, we spend the day feeling worried, sad, and angry. Sure, not every day can be great. We all have times when we feel left out, or we've been worrying about a big game or hard test, or something didn't go the way we had hoped. It isn't easy to feel good when your day feels tough.

An important part of feeling happy and content in all sorts of situations involves remembering the things you *do* have. In every situation, you have a secret weapon: you. You are kind, helpful, and funny, and you are learning more every day. You have people who love you and people who will always be there to help. On some blank paper or in a journal, take a few minutes to list:

- Three qualities, strengths, or talents you are most proud of
- Three people (pets can count too!) you love spending time with
- Three things you enjoy doing

Use the Challenging Worry Worksheet you downloaded to practice the E step, identifying thoughts, challenging negative thoughts, and choosing accurate and helpful ones.

Key Takeaways

In the moment, it seems like whatever thought pops up in our minds is just true. That's *just the situation we're in and that's all there is to it.* But there are a million things that are also true in every situation and maybe even more true. Remember, just because you thought it, doesn't mean you think it!

While we don't have the power to control others, or the world around us, we do have the power to control the direction and focus of our thoughts and, from there, our subsequent actions. Which means that we have the power to create our experience.

Focusing on the goal and knowing that you'll handle things as they come, rather than anticipating and preventing them, may be the fastest and easiest path to creating more of what you want.

The E step helps your child notice their thoughts or "self-talk" so that they can build self-awareness and be in a position to evaluate and choose their response.

- Identify self-talk:
    - Helpful or unhelpful?
    - Common warning messages from our bully.

- Challenge anxious and negative self-talk:
    - Challenge questions.
    - Choose your focus.

- Practice choosing accurate and helpful self-talk.

- Remember strengths: what I *do* have, what I *can* do.

We know that even our thinking becomes habit over time. Help your child become more aware of their habits or patterns of thinking by helping them list or write down their most common worry or sad thoughts.

CHAPTER 8

The A Step: Attitudes and Actions That Can Help

You gain strength, courage, and confidence by every experience in which you really stop to look fear in the face. You must do the thing you think you cannot do.

—Eleanor Roosevelt

We are often asked: "What is the one thing you'd like every parent to know?" and our answer is always, "When in doubt, encourage approach." Approach, as opposed to avoidance—of challenge, of fears, of the unknown—is the fastest and longest-lasting method of building self-confidence, adaptability, and resilience and reducing anxiety. Unfortunately, it can also be the hardest thing to do. It goes against every instinct to plan, prevent, and flee. It puts your child at risk for facing disappointment, heartache, loss, embarrassment, and/or discomfort. Yet it is what we recommend. It is also the piece that is left out of most books; even some counselors avoid it, ironically, because it is a challenge.

Approach versus Avoidance

When challenges arise, our instincts tell us to retreat. This happens in all types of circumstances, not just anxiety-provoking ones. We've discussed that when we're worried about an outcome, our instinct tells us to avoid the situation. For instance, if we're worried that we won't meet a deadline for a challenging project (like doing taxes), it's possible that we'll decide to start working on a less-challenging project without any deadline first (like cleaning out a closet)—it pushes off the "bad" feeling of stress and fear of failure or other negative outcome. This also happens when we are disappointed or saddened. Our instinct tells us to withdraw and give up. We've called this the "hibernation" instinct. When our body tells us *A cold long winter is approaching—there's nothing you can do about it, so conserve your resources, energy, and food, and just sleep. Don't talk to anyone or go anywhere—just hibernate.* For instance, if you've been rejected by someone you cared about, it's understandable that your first instinct is to think, *I'll never find a person like that again* or *I'm not attractive or* [fill in the positive adjective] *enough, so no one will ever fall in love with me,* and you might decide to stay home and watch Netflix that night (hibernate)—which pushes off the "bad" feelings of loss and loneliness. Those who have struggled with depression will know that the weight of the hibernation instinct is heavy. It's very difficult to feel like getting up when your body is so sure it wants to sleep.

When this happens, you can remind yourself that it's a false alarm (or a false winter storm warning) and remind yourself it's time to think of a more accurate and useful way to interpret the situation. But until you *do the thing* you've put off or avoided, you don't really feel much better, or learn anything new about these types of situations. If you've avoided or pushed off the negative feeling, you end up learning that things *are* really stressful and hard, and you're actually not capable of handling them. The "bad" feeling will continue to come in challenging situations and could even gain strength over time. If avoidance continues to develop as a pattern, you'll find yourself developing the narrative (your belief) that goes along with it—*I'm not good with deadlines, I'm a procrastinator, no one loves me*—and eventually develop an identity or self-definition of yourself as one who is alone, vulnerable, and incapable. Over time you can imagine how this can impact your self-confidence and reduce your ability to be resilient when things do go wrong, as they sometimes do.

While avoidance is usually the first instinct, it is also usually the "false" instinct—the one your alarm suggests, not the thing that will actually help in this situation. Approaching the challenge—making even the smallest move to tackle the difficult task (e.g., getting out of bed to take a shower), or taking the smallest step toward the uncomfortable feeling (calling an old friend or family member to get together)— will make you feel better. It gives you the opportunity to learn from the experience that you are capable, that challenges can be overcome, and heartache is temporary. Through a pattern of approach, we accumulate experiences of being strong and competent. Over time, we develop self-confidence and resilience in place of anxiety and hopelessness.

The A Step: Actions That Can Help

In every situation, how we react comes from a combination of our biology (physiological process), our thoughts (cognitive process), and our actions (behaviors). We are working to be in charge of our response, rather than reacting purely from instinct. In the F and E steps we addressed two of these factors. In the F step (What am I **F**eeling?) we built awareness of our fight-or-flight alarm system, physiological signs of anxiety, and understanding of what is happening in our bodies. In the E step (**E**xpecting bad things to happen?), we built awareness of our inner voice and our patterns of thinking so we can choose the most accurate and useful focus and interpretation of the situation instead of following the first thought that pops up.

The A step in the FEAR plan stands for **A**ttitudes and Actions that can help. This step is about choosing an action that is useful and then approaching things that are challenging rather than avoiding them. We want our kids to choose actions that will be most useful in getting them closer to their goal. Now that they are equipped with awareness of their patterns and of their physiological experience, and the ability to identify and challenge their negative thoughts, and they have the F and E steps to help walk them through the moment, we recommend encouraging and even creating opportunities for our kids to take on challenges or face new and uncomfortable experiences so they can practice the A step: choosing actions that will move them closer to their goal, rather than avoidance.

Planning Approach: Exposure and Behavioral Activation

How do we help our kids stop avoiding and start approaching challenges? We have learned, through many years of research and working with clients, that what we call *planning approach*, systematically, can be incredibly efficient in turning around even long-lived patterns of avoidance. Put simply, when challenges seem too big to overcome, it's a good idea to plan to approach the challenge in small steps. When you feel like you want to give up, and it feels like there's no point, it's a good idea to plan approach to social connections and meaningful actions. This makes sense—to develop resilience, it's necessary to experience overcoming fears, rejections, and losses.

You may have heard the term *exposure therapy* in movies or in the media. Exposure in this context is the clinical term used to describe a systematic practice of approaching challenges in real-world situations. It's unfortunate that the field has struggled to find a more friendly term for it that is catchy and captures the essence of the strategy—"exposure therapy" doesn't sound like something you'd want to sign up for, and it's often misrepresented. But it is incredibly effective in helping children (and adults) turn around old patterns of avoidance and turn off the false alarms. Many experts consider exposure the key component of effective therapies for anxiety. Approaching activities requiring energy, effort, and social connection is called *behavioral activation* and is also thought to be a key component for change for those struggling with depression. The principles behind these therapeutic strategies are relevant for everyone—not just those struggling with depression and anxiety.

The goal of these planned practices is to expose your child to feeling anxious in various situations so that they have opportunities to endure some distress and become comfortable and expert in using coping strategies—the FEAR plan. These practices allow their mind and body to learn something new. Without real-world experience, the body's natural instincts (alarm, avoidance, hibernation) will have difficulty shifting. Think of building a muscle—a muscle will not change without repeated use of the muscle in a new way, and this can be uncomfortable at first because it's not what the body is used to. Slowly, with repetition, the muscle will feel more comfortable doing the action. Our nervous system works very much in the same way. Our body's alarm response adjusts with repetition—a fight-or-flight alarm fades with practice of approaching something that we once avoided.

When introducing this idea to your child, here's the main concept to get across: Their body has learned to give false alarms in different situations. Anxiety or self-doubt makes it hard to see what's most likely to happen, and instead make us focus on the bad things that *might* happen. We have to train our body and mind to know that there's no danger and that we can handle all kinds of things. We do that by not avoiding the things or situations in which we feel uncomfortable.

Before you begin putting your child in new and difficult situations, it's helpful to explain the rationale for these practices. Sometimes giving an analogy, or even telling a personal story, can help communicate the rationale for exposure tasks to kids. You can describe a time when you were anxious about going somewhere or doing something, but after a few times it got easier.

Therapists often use the analogy of anxiety as a bully: What if a bully says he's going to beat you up if you don't give him your lunch money? What will happen if you give him your lunch money? He'd leave you alone right away because he got what he wanted. But what will happen the next day? He'll probably come back, right? Anxiety works that way too. If you do what it says, it comes back—even stronger. What could you do so that the bully would stop bothering you? If you didn't give him your lunch money, what might happen? Well, he might get angry, but what if you still didn't give it to him? And then the next day you still didn't give him your lunch money? Pretty soon he'd leave you alone and try to get what he wants from someone else. Anxiety can be the bully. With anxiety, if it says *Don't ask your friend to come over because she'll make fun of you,* what could you do to make the anxiety leave you alone and stop telling you there's danger? Right! Ask your friend to come over! Then the next time, the anxiety would bother you less about asking a friend over.

CONVERSATION STARTER   Remember that when you are in fight-or-flight mode, your body is designed to run from danger. As you've learned, when a worry pops up and your alarm goes off, you usually start thinking of ways to make sure the "bad" thing you're worrying about doesn't happen. You might even try to avoid it in some way. If you avoid or run away from a challenge, your body learns that the situation really is dangerous.

When you listen to your worries and try to avoid a "bad" thing from happening, you don't learn that:

- The "bad" thing wasn't going to happen.
- Even if things don't turn out perfectly, you can handle it.

By avoiding, your only experience is that you couldn't handle it, and it really was dangerous. The good news is that if you choose to face the difficult situation, taking it on instead of avoiding it, your body learns that the situation is not dangerous and that you can handle it. Only then does your alarm stop going off as often as it once did, and the worries stop popping up and bothering you so much.

To teach your worry that things are really okay, you have to do the thing you've been avoiding and show your worry that you can handle it. For example, if you have been avoiding sitting with other kids at lunch, you could plan to sit with another kid who may also be sitting alone. If you have been avoiding raising your hand in class, you could plan to raise your hand in your favorite class when there is a question that you know the answer to.

The actions you choose are very important, because they create the experiences you have today. When trying to decide what to do when you're feeling worried or anxious, keep in mind these tips:

- Do the thing that will most likely lead you to your end goal.

- Do the opposite of what worry wants you to do.

Example: "Doing the thing" means taking a small step toward your end goal. Let's practice what doing the thing means. What would be an action that could lead a kid closer to their end goal?

Luke wants to be a good swimmer, but he has been worried that he might not be able to pass the swim test. So he has been avoiding getting in the pool during his swim lessons.

Worry action: Sit on the bench during swim lessons → Experience: I can't handle swim class; I'm not a good swimmer.

Do the thing: What are some possibilities you can think of?

The actions that come from worry or fear are usually actions that avoid the situation or try to prevent anything bad from happening.

Try doing the opposite of what worry tells you. For example, if your worry says, *Don't raise your hand!* the opposite would be to raise your hand. If it says, *Don't say hi!* doing the opposite would be to say hi to the person you were thinking of. If you are afraid to sleep alone at night, your worry would say, *Ask Mom or Dad to sleep with you,* and doing the opposite would be to tell them to check on you after twenty minutes but not stay.

Gradual and Repeated Approach

Approaching a challenge in small steps, rather than all at once, usually works best. It's easier for a person to approach a small challenge than a big one—their alarm will be less heightened, and they might think it's more likely they'll have success—so they'll be more likely to agree to do it and more likely to have an experience of successful approach. Their body still learns the lesson that the thing they were avoiding was not dangerous and they could handle it, so it's still a very big and useful step.

For planning approach, we try to think of small steps to make it easier and more likely for your child to have success. Take the feared thing or situation—social situations, performance situations, or just uncomfortable feelings—and break it up into all of the ways that it is challenging, then practice approaching each component a little bit at a time. Planning repeated practice is also crucial because it allows your child's body to get used to the discomfort, and then eventually the alarm fades. In other words, the more you do it, the easier it gets. We know that something is easier if

- It has been done before (*familiarity*: for example, playing a sport I've played many times before).

- There is *support* (for example, a friend is going too, versus going without knowing anyone else).

- The *duration* is relatively short (say, one hour of a new activity versus a full day at a new camp versus staying overnight).

- The territory is familiar (*distance*: in the backyard versus in the neighborhood versus in a different city).

- The degree of *difficulty* of the task is less (for example, playing a sport I feel confident about in my yard versus playing a sport I don't feel confident about in front of a large crowd).

Once your child has taken the easy steps and repeated them a few times, they will be ready to take on the more difficult steps. Something that would have been a major challenge—looming as the hardest thing you could ever do—will seem less difficult after you've practiced the smaller steps. We like to say that fear is like a house of cards; if you take one or two cards out from the bottom, the whole thing collapses! In planning stages, start with listing the steps in order of difficulty, from least to most difficult. In clinical terms we call this *making a hierarchy*; for working with the FEAR plan, we call it a FEAR ladder. You can use My Practice Ladder (available for download at (http://www.newharbinger. com/46967) to plan out the order of steps to practice with your child.

Here's an example: if you're planning a practice for your child who is afraid of dogs, the first practice should not be going to a dog park. First, there will be some dogs at the park that are running off-leash, and some may be more rambunctious than you'd want for the first practice. Second, multiple dogs would be more difficult for your child than just one dog. A dog park might be better as a practice after several practices with a single dog. So you begin with a single dog practice, and first break it down to the components of the fear.

What if the dog jumps on me? Practice sitting in the same room with a dog on a leash but far enough away that the dog can't reach you. Do this a few times, and notice that dogs may jump for the first few minutes, then get bored and lose interest. Then sit closer to the dog.

What if the dog bites me? Let the dog smell your hand. Keep doing that for ten minutes. Then pat the dog for ten seconds. Then repeat.

Now your child may be ready for sitting in the room with the dog off the leash. Continue from there.

Come up with practices that will be easy to plan, easy to control the outcomes, and easy to repeat.

Types of Practices:

- *Overcoming a fear*—speaking in front of others, being away overnight, being outside where there might be bees

- *Solving a problem*—facing a bully, getting along with a sibling, resolving a friendship issue, confronting someone

- *Preparing for an upcoming event*—a big test, game, or performance coming up, a social event

- *Learning a new skill*—learning an instrument, playing a sport, learning something new in art class or school

- *Completing a task*—finishing homework, submitting an assignment, presenting a speech, playing a piece of music

- *Achieving something*—getting a role in a performance, getting onto a sports team

- *Being the boss of our feelings*—angry with a teacher or parent or friend, scared of making mistakes

When thinking of approach practices, it's important to keep these tips in mind:

- *The practice is carried out in a gradual way.* With gradual exposure, not only can children habituate to anxiety-provoking situations, but they can also build their confidence in applying their coping strategies and experience a sense of mastery.

- *The child will experience some anxiety when practicing their skills,* but this is to be expected and it is okay. The more they practice facing these situations, the less anxious they will feel.

- *The aim is not to remove anxiety* but to practice being able to manage it.

- *Depending on the exposure task, the child may need to stay in the situation for a certain amount of time.* If they get out of the situation too quickly, then they haven't experienced that they can cope.

- *The FEAR steps need to be practiced repeatedly.* The more your child practices them, the more automatic they will become.

Here are the steps for each exposure task:

1. Review the fear hierarchy and discuss the exposure task.

2. Plan and role-play parts of the exposure task.

3. Review the FEAR plan.

4. Complete the exposure task; wait for the anxiety to go down, and don't allow avoidance.

5. If it's too hard, ask what they *can* do.

6. Review and reward for effort.

7. Plan the next practice.

CONVERSATION STARTER: EXAMPLE LADDER Jill, a sixth-grader, worried so much about school that she had not been to school for several weeks! Because tackling a worry this big at one time can be very hard, Jill found it much easier to break her worry into steps. She returned to school by first sitting in the main office in the mornings. After a few days, she went to just her first class. After that, she stayed for her second class. A few days later, she could stay at school all the way through lunch.

Taking things a step at a time worked great for Jill. At each step, she saw that the things she feared did not happen. And she realized that if there was a little challenge at school, like a tough test or a mean classmate, she could handle it. Seeing that she could handle one step increased her confidence about handling the next step. Before she knew it, Jill was back to spending the entire day at school.

Let's make a plan for new, difficult, or uncomfortable situations that you want to worry less about. We'll make the list go from easiest to hardest.

Now pick one of those situations. Then, using the ladder (My Practice Ladder, available for download at http://www.newharbinger.com/46967), break it into five small, more manageable steps. At the bottom of the ladder, put the easiest step. At the top of the ladder, put your hardest step. For each step, write down the days on which you will tackle these steps. This will keep you moving up your ladder to your ultimate goal! Here is Jill's ladder as an example.

Jill's Practice Ladder: Worry about going to school

Step 5 (hardest): Stay at school for full day.

Days I will do this step: November 24, 28, 29

Step 4: Stay at school for morning class, lunch, and recess.

Days I will do this step: November 21, 22, 23

Step 3: Stay at school until lunchtime.

Days I will do this step: November 15, 16, 17

Step 2: Go to my first class.

Days I will do this step: November 10, 12, 14

Step 1 (easiest): Go into school and sit in main office for twenty minutes.

Days I will do this step: November 7, 8, 9

You can use your Practice Ladder for any worry. Think of other worries you want to tackle but feel are overwhelming. For each of these worries, build a ladder. Your ladder does not have to have five steps. If five steps seems overwhelming, make a longer ladder—you can make seven steps or even ten steps.

Tackle one worry ladder at a time. Give yourself a few days at each step to get used to that experience, to see that nothing bad happens, and to show yourself that you can cope with whatever comes your way. Keep moving up your ladder to reach your ultimate goal! And don't forget to reward yourself for a job well done. When Jill reached her goal of staying at school for the full day, her mom and dad took her out to her favorite pizza place for dinner!

Change doesn't happen overnight—it takes time and practice. Review and plan for the next week. After each practice, review the FEAR hierarchy and discuss which exposure tasks should come next.

As we have mentioned, even though there is only one chapter in this book that is dedicated to exposure, we recommend and encourage you to spend several weeks on this practice.

We recommend at least four weeks of practice for each difficulty or type of fear.

Don't Become Part of Their Worry Cycle: Limit Accommodation

Your parental instinct to protect is usually spot on. In most situations, this natural effort to protect works just fine. But often parents slip into protecting their kids from negative emotions, which is not always the instinct to follow. Protecting your child from emotional distress can backfire. In the case of a child who experiences anxiety false alarms often, this natural instinct clearly isn't the one to follow. In the case of anxiety, in particular, being overly vigilant in relieving your child's anxiety can end up serving to *maintain* the anxiety rather than relieving it.

Take the example of a child who is worried before getting on a plane for the first time. This is a natural and typical experience of anxiety— our bodies weren't designed to fly, so our primitive brains definitely go into fight-or-flight in anticipation of it. Your natural first instinct might be to explain all the reasons why flying on a plane is safe. "There are thousands of flights every day; traveling on a plane is safer than traveling in a car! I have traveled for twenty years and been on countless planes, and you see I've never had a problem. There are lots of people working to make sure we are safe. The pilots know what they are doing. I wouldn't take you if I didn't think it was safe..." Providing a *little* bit of data might be effective in convince most kids to approach and experience their first flight. But for kids who get stuck in a worry cycle, whose alarm has gone off and is not satisfied with data—asking you to explain the news story about the crash last month and how you can guarantee no germs on the seat—the data and reassurance of safety actually ends up feeding the worry cycle. You might not think it, but this actually feeds into the sense that this situation is dangerous.

Reassurance is one of the most common forms of avoidance that parents can get sucked into offering unintentionally. When a child describes what they're worried about, it's natural for a parent to give reassurance. Sometimes we do this almost automatically. For example, if they ask "What if you get sick? Who would take care of me?" you might respond, "Don't worry, I'm healthy, I won't get sick!" But if we spend too much time giving reassurance, we're actually feeding the anxiety. Rather than having to make sure that things are okay, it's more effective to help the child identify the thought as a worry and get bored with it. Remember, trying to make sure things are okay works almost like avoidance: it may provide short-term relief, but makes it worse in the long run.

Think of the example of a child who is worried about monsters under the bed. We might say, "Don't worry, there are no monsters under your bed—why don't you check under the bed and check in your closet and see?" But suggesting they check validates that there's a reason to be worried. The child might wonder if they missed checking somewhere important! Similarly, reassurance validates that there's a reason to be worried. Rather than suggesting checking under the bed, what if you suggested that it's a false alarm? "It's just a false alarm—there's no such thing as monsters. They're just make-believe, so no one needs to check or worry." Similarly, rather than saying, "Don't worry, I'm healthy" (which, over time, will require them to keep checking the status of your health), it's better to say, "See, the anxiety alarm is going off at the wrong time. Let's pay attention to what we want to be thinking about right now instead."

In cases where you're not sure—wondering if you should explain things in more detail and explain nuances or risks—instead of getting sucked into the cycle by providing reassurance, we recommend using the *one-time rule*. If you really feel your child doesn't understand something, or doesn't have all of the information they need to make a good choice, and it's an opportunity to provide your perspective on a new topic (such as what you think about plane travel), absolutely communicate your knowledge and your values—once. Explain everything you know, answer their questions, and communicate what you think about it in depth— one time. After that, keep it short and consistent. "We know it's scary, we know it's uncomfortable the first time—your body just hasn't learned that it's safe yet—it's new and different. But we'll keep at it and teach your body that you're okay." When they ask again, be even more brief— "Your body is feeling uncomfortable, but you can remind your body that it's just new and different, not dangerous"—and then keep packing. Or "The uncomfortable feelings will come and go, I know, but you'll be able to handle it," and keep moving toward the airport. Same response to all of their questions. Instead of trying to reassure them with specifics—like the data on air travel safety or how likely or unlikely problems are with air travel, which feeds anxiety—approach the challenge and keep reassurance low. This will speed both your child's approach of the challenging situation and the relief from their anxiety. This is why we recommend that you help your child approach their fears rather than help them relieve their fears.

Helping children relieve their own distress, or helping them avoid feeling bad, can counterproductively lead to their feeling less confident and more insecure, and may even stunt their natural development of coping skills. We want you to do less coping for your child and instead create opportunities for them to approach discomfort. Approaching the discomfort is more effective in the long term in relieving emotional distress than avoiding the discomfort. A lifestyle of choosing *approach* to discomfort over *avoidance* can replace anxiety with anticipation of new and challenging experiences for a lifetime.

We use the term *accommodation* for the ways in which parents modify routines or expectations to alleviate a child's distress or anxiety (see Kagan, Frank, & Kendall, 2017). Examples of accommodation include changing family activities so that the child can avoid discomfort or a feared situation, or providing reassurance (Thompson-Hollands et al., 2014b). Although a parent may think that accommodating helps make things easier, it actually makes things harder! Anything parents do to reduce discomfort might help in the short term, but making things easier for your child actually maintains the anxiety in the long run. A large body of research has established that accommodation contributes to the development and maintenance of anxiety in youth. Perhaps because parents think accommodation helps, it is common: in several studies, parents of youth with anxiety and parents of youth with OCD reported engaging in accommodating behavior (see Lebowitz et al., 2014; Flessner et al., 2011; Settipani & Kendall, 2017; Thompson-Hollands et al., 2014a, 2014b). Two aspects of accommodation have emerged: participation in the youth's symptoms (e.g. checking the weather for a child afraid of storms, buying new socks that feel "just right") and modification of family routines to avoid triggers (such as cancelling plans because a child will be anxious; Flessner et al., 2011; Lebowitz et al., 2013). Both types of accommodation are common, with the majority of parents reporting that they provide some kind of accommodation at least once a day (Flessner et al., 2011; Peris, Bergman, Langley, Chang, McCracken, & Piacentini, 2008).

Studies have also found that more frequent accommodation is associated with more severe symptoms and impairment at home and at school (Lebowitz et al., 2013). In addition, parents report negative results when they do *not* accommodate, such as the child becoming more anxious, or angry or abusive (Lebowitz et al., 2013). Although accommodation may negatively affect the child's autonomy and functioning, parents may accommodate because they lack other strategies. The FEAR plan is an alternate strategy.

Adopting a Lifestyle of Approach

Your family will need to make a bit of a lifestyle change to create an environment that supports approach. When a child experiences distress from anxiety, change the language. Your typical pattern may be to try to reassure, provide a back-up plan, or start coping *for* the child. Instead, try using new language, communicating confidence in their ability to tolerate a bad feeling or the fight-or-flight feeling that may have come when they were trying something new. Here are a few specific suggestions:

- Restate and acknowledge (show empathy) without providing reassurance or apologizing or getting into problem solving: "It sounds like the alarm is going off really loud right now" or "I can see it feels really bad to feel so uncomfortable."

- Communicate confidence: "It's tough, but you're tougher," "I'm not sure, but I bet you can handle whatever happens," or "The worry is saying all the things it usually says; you know what to do with it."

- Keep it short: "Why don't we wait and find out when we get there?" or "We won't know until we go."

- Communicate your values and expectations: "It's really important that we go [try, handle responsibilities, show our support, and so on]."

- Set limits and give an opportunity to approach: "We'll need to finish before we can go home, but I'll give you a minute to get things going."

With this lifestyle, your child can practice as part of a general goal to try new things, not just to face a specific challenge. For instance, planning to try a new food or planning to talk with new people, visiting new places, and trying new activities. Being in the habit of pushing past their comfort zone gives them a head start on building resilience.

Key Takeaways

If you've avoided negative feelings, you end up learning that things are really stressful and hard, and you're not capable of handling them. The "bad" feeling will continue to come in situations where there is challenge, and it could even gain strength over time.

If avoidance continues to develop as a pattern, you'll find yourself developing the narrative (your belief) that goes with it and eventually develop an identity or self-definition as alone, vulnerable, and incapable. Over time, this could reduce your self-confidence and resiliency when things do go wrong.

Approach to challenges, to fears, to the unknown—as opposed to avoidance of them—is the fastest and longest-lasting method of building self-confidence, adaptability, and resilience, and reducing anxiety.

The A step is about choosing a useful action and then approaching things that are challenging rather than avoiding them.

When your child is trying to decide what to do when feeling worried or anxious, they should keep in mind these tips:

- Do the thing that will most likely lead you to your goal.

- Do the opposite of what worry wants you to do.

When planning approach, think of small steps to make it easier and more likely for your child to have success. Take the feared thing or situation and break it up into all aspects of the challenge and practice approaching each, one at a time.

When thinking of approach practices, it's important to keep these tips in mind:

- The practice is carried out in a gradual way. With gradual exposure, not only can children habituate to anxiety-provoking situations, but they can also build their confidence in applying their coping strategies and experience a sense of mastery.

- The child will experience some anxiety when practicing their skills, but this is to be expected, and it is okay. The more they practice facing these situations the less anxious they will feel.

- The aim is not to remove anxiety but to practice being able to manage it.

- Depending on the challenge they are approaching, the child may need to stay in the situation for a certain amount of time. If they get out of the situation too quickly, then they haven't experienced that they can cope, which can interfere with building a sense of mastery.

- The FEAR steps need to be practiced repeatedly. The more your child practices them, the more automatic they will become.

There are also activities in our book, The Worry Workbook for Kids (Khanna & Ledley, 2019) and in our online program for kids, "Camp Cope-A-Lot" (Kendall & Khanna, 2008) that can provide opportunities for even more practice.

CHAPTER 9

The R Step: Results and Rewards

If one advances confidently in the direction of his dreams, and endeavors to live the life which he has imagined, he will meet with a success unexpected in common hours.

—Henry David Thoreau

So far, through teaching and practicing the F, E, and A steps, your child has gained awareness: able to identify when they are feeling stressed, anxious, or down. They have begun to develop the habit of thinking about what they are thinking, or what they are expecting to happen when they notice that their alarm has been set off. They've learned the benefits of deep breathing and of attending to the present. They are practicing staying in the mind-set of learning, growth, and progress rather than success and failure. They have planned to use their new skills to practice facing challenges and to start a lifetime of approach rather than avoidance. Each of these skills, if rewarded consistently, is more likely to be associated with positive feeling; this makes it more likely your child will repeat and use these skills in more and more new and complex situations. This is the focus of the R step, the last step of the FEAR plan. **R**esults and Rewards reminds them to learn from results and to reward themselves for taking the actions and attitudes that helped get them closer to their goals. Behaviors that are followed by reward are more likely to be repeated. It's such a simple maxim, but we can't overemphasize how powerful it can be in creating lasting changes in patterns of behavior and thought.

R: Results and Rewards

The R step reminds us to reward our efforts, not our outcomes. A reward can give us a needed push when the effort feels hard and also helps teach us that doing tough things can be uncomfortable at first but feels really good in the end. Behavior that is followed by a reward (anything that makes your kid feel good) is likely to be practiced again in the future. We want our kids to keep trying, which is why we strongly advise rewarding every form of approach. We want them to feel good about trying and to know that their parent(s)/loved ones are proud of them when they try, even when it doesn't turn out as they had hoped. We can even plan rewards in advance so that when they approach the difficult situations, regardless of the outcome, they are rewarded for their efforts.

Before getting into the specifics of reward and reinforcement, let's discuss the importance of setting realistic and appropriate goals and expectations and evaluating performance or actions fairly, with perspective, and with compassion.

Self-Evaluation

All of us, both kids and adults, tend to rely on outside sources for a sense of achievement—like needing a friend to compliment us before feeling good about ourselves. We also tend to reward ourselves infrequently, and only for performance we deem satisfactory, rather than for the attempt. It is as if we think we don't deserve praise unless we have made no mistakes. With such extraordinary standards, it's almost impossible to feel confident when attempting anything challenging.

Further, kids often set a very short timeline for themselves to learn and master new things and set high expectations about outcomes that aren't 100 percent in their control. Having goals is important, but if expectations are to achieve outcomes that are out of your control and without error, they will likely fuel fear and disappointment.

In the R step, we encourage kids to evaluate their results with an eye on all the facts, with perspective, and with compassion.

CONVERSATION STARTER The R step is the last step of the FEAR plan. So far, we've talked about knowing what you're feeling (F) inside and ignoring any false alarms. Then we talked about making sure what you're thinking is really the most useful to be thinking (the E step) and not focusing on just all the bad things that might happen. And we've been trying to practice planning to do difficult things instead of avoiding them (the A step). The R step in the FEAR plan is the one where you remember to be proud of yourself and to reward yourself for practicing—even if you took just a small step. Any step toward helping yourself feel better or doing something that was difficult is a win.

Often we set really high expectations—for ourselves and even for what other people should do. I still do that sometimes [insert example, such as finding the perfect birthday gift for a friend and then the friend loving the gift or making good shots and winning a basketball game]. It's really easy to feel disappointed if things don't go as easily as you wanted or didn't turn out exactly as you would have liked. But we're all still just learning and growing. No one is perfect. Instead of getting too disappointed or frustrated with myself, I have to remind myself that I am still working on [getting to be a better basketball player, or realizing there is no such thing as a "perfect" gift—all gifts are perfect, because they come from wanting to show someone your appreciation], and I'm human—I make mistakes, get tired, and am not at my best all the time. And so many things go into what happens in the end that I can't measure myself on that. We can only control what we do and not what happens outside or what other people do [other people might be really strong players; the other person might not like to read books, and I thought they did]. But I try to stay proud that I [got out there and played and learn from the experience] [found out that my friend doesn't like to read, but does like something else]. [sports: The more I play, the better I get, and I can feel good that I'm working hard and trying to help out my team—we might even win some games along the way] [gift: I'm glad I did something to show my appreciation of my friend, and another time I might pick a gift they really like!]

Any step toward trying something new or doing something challenging is something to feel proud of. Sometimes the result might not be perfect—you might not come in first place—but just practicing and putting in time and putting yourself out there to do something that's challenging makes you a winner in my book. You deserve to be proud of yourself for thinking through your FEAR plan.

Let's say you made a plan to hang out with some friends—you decide to focus on being a good friend to them, and you plan things you can do to show kindness rather than focusing on whether or not they are liking you. When you get to your friend's house, you were kind and good at taking turns and listening to their opinions. But your friend wasn't that nice, or you ended up not having that much fun. You can reward yourself for being a good friend, and I'd be really proud of you for focusing on what you could do to be a good friend and not getting too focused on what didn't go as well as you would have liked.

Self-Reward

The R step also helps to encourage kids to reward themselves, rather than waiting for someone else's judgment or a specific outcome. We've learned that rewards or praise help us push ourselves when the effort feels hard and learn that doing things that are tough can be uncomfortable at first but feels really good in the end. Encourage your child to feel proud of efforts and accomplishments. Ask them to describe a situation in which they felt proud of themself. Point out how someone (a celebrity, book character, or athlete) talked about feeling proud because they did something challenging, even if the outcome wasn't ideal.

CONVERSATION STARTER   It's great to plan something fun or nice to look forward to after doing something difficult. When you're trying to use the FEAR plan, plan a nice reward for yourself for putting in the effort to do something challenging.

Any time you put in effort, or try, to use the FEAR plan in a difficult situation, you should plan to reward yourself. I can also help get rewards ready for you—I also want to encourage you and reward you when you *decide* to try and when you *try* to help yourself with a challenge.

Be ready to reward, both for practicing the FEAR plan and for actions that show a sense of independence, confidence, and character in your child's real experience. For example, praise heartily for the thoughtfulness of and effort in baking a cake for Dad's birthday, even though it came out a little burnt.

Rewarding Process, Not Outcome

Parents also must keep focused on rewarding the process—like trying something new, preparing for an event, practicing a skill, asking questions, attempting to problem solve—and not the outcome. Improvement, not perfection, is the goal. Praise persistence, problem solving, creativity, teamwork, purpose—praise getting better at these. Even praise *failure*! "It's so great that you tried this really hard thing." "I'm so proud of you; you worked so hard, and you're getting better every time."

We always want to reward any type of approach, even if it's just a small part of the task, or things don't go exactly as planned. Again, learning theory tells us that the environment and the consequences of our experiences are constantly shaping our view of ourselves and our world. We want our kids to learn that moving toward a challenge, even if they don't get the outcome they wanted, feels good. It's what's behind the saying "Just as long as you try your best" but doesn't demand to know whether it is actually their *best*—which is always hard to quantify! We assume that kids want to do their best, always, but it's hard to master something new and to approach difficult things, and it's especially hard when fear or self-doubt get in the way. We also don't want to withhold praise or convey disappointment when things don't go well, because your child then learns that not gaining the outcome they wanted is dangerous, and they might want to avoid pursuing challenges. We want to convey that we are okay with imperfect outcomes as long as their efforts keep them moving toward their goals.

Try to communicate the importance of *approach* (or moving toward a goal) and not just a specific external *outcome* in everyday situations, too, not just when you're your child is practicing the FEAR plan. We know this can be tough. There may be a time when a poor test grade might impact a semester grade or even the entire school year grade, and you may have anxiety *yourself* about whether your child will achieve the goals you think they are capable of. It's a good opportunity to remind them that they are still learning and growing. That no one is perfect. That it's time to focus on what they learned and what they might do differently next time, and that they can be proud of their trying and learning from the experience. The more they approach the challenge, the easier it will get, and the more likely they will be to one day have the outcome they are hoping for.

You may find yourself asking, "What grade did you get on the test?" "Did you get the part in the play?" or "Did you win the game?" rather than asking "Did you try out?" or "You worked really hard on that project this weekend, did you present it at school today?" Nothing wrong with setting high standards, but if you don't reward the process of trying and approaching the challenge—if you don't let them know that reaching a goal involves successes *and* failures along the way—your child may miss out on a sense of satisfaction and be in an almost endless state of tension and stress. The time to reward is as soon as the attempt has been made, or even during preparation, not after they achieve the "right" outcome. For example, if your child is studying for a big test, praise the time spent studying or finishing the homework, instead of waiting to reward the good grade.

Types of Rewards

Rewards don't need to be tangible (like a toy or a food treat)—an "I'm so proud of you for trying," a pat on the back, a smile, a hug, acknowledging their strengths, all lead to good feelings. These are strong rewards. Sometimes the reward is built in—when you do something that you may have avoided, you end up getting the benefit of doing it. For example, let's say you have been avoiding speaking to new people. A challenge might be ordering ice cream at an unfamiliar or new store, and the reward is built in—they get the ice cream *and* the good feeling that comes from doing something new *without* letting worry stop them. You can prompt your child to make a list of rewards, such as fun activities they can plan, nice things they can say to themselves, or a privilege or small prize they can earn. (You can download a Ways I Can Reward Myself worksheet at http://www.newharbinger.com/46967.)

Some of the parents we have worked with have created reward jars in which they put sticky notes with a variety of small rewards, such as "favorite dessert" or "15 minutes of extra computer time." Their child can pull one from the jar at the end of each task or at the end of the day. The actual reward may come later, but the acknowledgment of the reward is prompt.

Some parents struggle with the idea of rewards, thinking it is a bribe. The idea is not to bribe your child (*If you say hi to someone new, you'll get a toy*) but rather to reward your child for effort (*I like how brave you were when you said hi to Sam*).

Parents often ask if they'll have to give rewards *forever*. The answer is no. As your child becomes confident in using the FEAR plan and developing a habit of approach, you won't have to plan specific rewards—but you should continue to provide encouragement, recognition, and support. Attention and praise are powerful rewards that you can and should use long term.

A note of caution: Stay away from punishment when it comes to working on coping and confidence, and try not to use withholding or taking away a reward as a punishment, either. Some family traditions include punishment for misbehavior. We don't want to debate the larger costs of such an approach here, but we believe that punishment is not the best way to encourage good behavior. Punishment may stop the behavior you don't like, but it may also stunt your child's capacity for resilient and confident behavior. Praise of reward for effort will far outperform any attempts to encourage resilience using punishment. Change the family tradition, and reward for trying!

Keep Your Praise-to-Criticism Ratio High

Praise and acknowledgment are perhaps a parent's most powerful tools in shaping their child's behaviors. A simple shift to praising more than criticizing can guide them away from developing self-doubt and toward developing self-confidence. Here are some things you can do to keep the ratio of praise to criticism high:

- Even when you know something can be improved, rather than first pointing out the mistakes, point out what was done well.

- Vary the focus of your praise—acknowledge not just academic or athletic success but also good character traits (when your child is thoughtful, helpful, supportive, funny, honest, responsible, a good friend).

- When they're being good, let them know you notice.

Check In On Yourself: Are You Ready?

Make sure you're okay with giving the reward—and also with the option to not give any particular reward. You don't want to offer inviting a friend to sleep over if you're not comfortable with having that friend over. For rewards to work, you'll have to say it, mean it, and do it. If you've offered a reward and your child has done the task, it's essential that you follow through. Not following through undermines the potency of rewards, and future reward plans will be ineffective.

Components of Successful Rewards

Reward effort, if not success.

Plan ahead so you know what will be rewarded and what the rewards will be.

Selecting rewards that are desirable by your child.

Deliver rewards promptly.

> Be consistent.
>
> Say it, mean it, do it.

Setting Limits Is Okay

Sometimes it is important to set limits for anxious youth. If your child is having a tantrum, even if it is in an effort to avoid anxiety, it's important to set a limit and stand by it. Anxiety doesn't force us to break rules or speak rudely to others or throw tantrums—it's okay to set limits. But, as with rewards, it's important to be consistent. For example, if a child has a tantrum in the morning when they have to get ready for school, and then they get to stay home instead of going to school late, that will reinforce morning tantrums. Don't feel guilty or bad about setting limits for your anxious child—consistent limit setting and predictable responses help give children a sense of stability and security.

Of course, you should be setting age-appropriate expectations, using clear and polite commands, and offering calm notices that give your child a chance to comply. Don't go overboard; don't give unnecessary commands. Often the fastest way to make a behavior stop is to ignore it. Young children may engage in silly behavior that can disappear when ignored.

Principles of Reinforcement

Psychology has long recognized and studied the merits of rewards. Research indicates that those who know the principles behind rewarding behavior are better at implementing rewards. So let's take a stroll through the basic principles that guide the psychology of rewards.

In behavioral psychology, or behaviorism, rewards are also called *positive reinforcement*. The goal of positive reinforcement is to increase the likelihood of a desired behavior. For example, if you'd like your child to say "excuse me" and wait instead of interrupting, then you'd want to praise him every time he says "excuse me" and waits.

Behaviorism has also identified that positive reinforcement can also reinforce behaviors you *don't* want to see. Like when your child displays anxiety and you hug or hold them, or give them a chance to avoid (which is what they want), you are inadvertently reinforcing the undesirable behavior. When your child complains and gets you to focus your attention on them and engage with them, it will actually increase how long and how often they complain.

Ignoring a behavior will be more effective in reducing that behavior. When you see behaviors that you don't like, ignore it or remove your attention. This doesn't means you ignore your child when they are managing anxiety and coping; rather, you can use attention as a reward. This experience communicates that they get your attention by being able to cope.

Now that your child has the basics of the FEAR plan, they are ready to begin practicing using the steps in real-world situations, starting with some planned practice. Remember, all along the way you want to reward effort and attitude. Do not accommodate anxiety and avoidance. Reward the many little steps, even if it's a long walk.

Key Takeaways

The R step reminds your child to learn from results and to reward themself for taking the actions and attitudes that helped get them closer to their goals.

Behaviors that are followed by reward are more likely to be repeated.

- Recognize the importance of effort and attitude, rather than outcome.

- Work with your child to generate a reward list.

- Consistency is key.

- Keep the praise-to-criticism ratio high.

- Use praise and attention that is associated with a behavior you want (e.g., facing challenges, trying new things, friendliness, loyalty, etc.).

- Praise immediately and often.

- Identify and praise the process that leads to success, not the outcome.

- Reward for effort and even for partial success. The message is that your child can try challenging things and is able to cope with the challenges.

- It's okay to set age-appropriate expectations and limits.

PART 3

Serving Suggestions

CHAPTER 10

Putting It All Together

Success is not final, failure is not fatal: it is the courage to continue that counts.

—Winston Churchill

We started off this book with a promise to communicate the steps to giving your child the gift of resilience—the ability to respond adaptively in times of adversity so they can approach life with calm and confidence. We promised to not just offer a list of helpful tips and strategies, but also to explain the principles behind the strategies so that you can feel empowered to apply and adapt as you see fits best for your child.

We started with the premise that developing resilience requires three major ingredients: (1) awareness of and compassion for one's own emotional and physiological experience and patterns, (2) cultivating a mind-set of growth and flexibility, and (3) living with the intention to approach new and even uncomfortable situations and challenges, rather than to avoid or prevent them. To guide your child in building this foundation, we walked you through how to teach the FEAR plan—an easily remembered acronym that helps kids walk through the steps of being aware of their inner experience, being in charge of and choosing their thought and emotional process, and practicing approach over avoidance as often as possible. Though this is more of a lifestyle than a cure, and though there will be many highs and lows, setbacks and gains as they grow, we feel confident that with this understanding in hand, your child, regardless of their situation, can face any situation without feeling at a loss. They'll know that they have the ability to keep things in perspective, to adapt, to problem solve—in other words, to be resilient.

We hope that since you began this journey you've noticed that as a parent you are more frequently sharing your values rather than your fears, accepting both good and bad emotions as normal, modeling and encouraging putting things into perspective, and being a cheerleader more often than a bodyguard or a judge as your child charts their destiny. We also hope you've adopted a lifestyle of approach for yourself and your family, and that through your communication and your actions you're now modeling focus on what you can control and what you do have, and moving with purpose toward creating more of what you want.

We know how many things you are trying to do for the well-being of your child and family and how challenging it all is. If you reflect on what you haven't done or couldn't do, please do so with compassion, and not for too long. We are psychologists who do this for a living, and even we struggle to implement the principles every time. We are all "perfectly imperfect," but because we come from love and genuine intent to support, encourage, and appreciate our children, we can be confident that things will turn out just fine.

Using the FEAR Plan

To help your child see how the steps of the FEAR plan fit together, it's helpful to spend some time practicing using the FEAR plan in staged or preplanned scenarios and then ongoing as future events arise.

CONVERSATION STARTER You have learned how to slow down and listen to your thoughts, to check to see whether they are useful and whether you're focusing on the most helpful things. You've started planning on doing things that are new or uncomfortable instead of putting them off or avoiding them completely. The more you practice challenging anxious and sad thoughts, staying focused on what is really important, and doing more things that you've been putting off, the less your alarm will go off. The next time you notice your alarm going off, or you are feeling more anxious, sad, or mad than you think you need to, or for longer than you'd like, remember that you have a superpower. You can choose your focus and your next actions. Use the FEAR plan to help you remember how:

What Am I **F**eeling?

Spot the false alarm. The situation is not dangerous—it's just new, difficult, and uncomfortable.

Expecting Bad Things to Happen?

Identify your first thought, then challenge it.

Choose the most accurate and helpful thought. Ask yourself, *Is what I am thinking accurate? Is what I am thinking useful?* If it seems like you are spending too much time thinking about these thoughts, then it's probably not useful. Ask yourself, *What is most likely to happen?* If it's a situation you've faced before, recall what actually happened. Figure out the most important things to focus on. Remember that the bad things we worry about don't usually happen. Remember that you've successfully handled other new, uncomfortable, or unfamiliar situations before. Don't forget to remember how much you do have and how much you can do.

Attitudes and Actions that can help

Choose an action that will get you closer to your goal rather than avoiding the challenge. Remember what you can control: your thoughts and your actions.

Choose an action that will most likely lead to your goal. Do the opposite of what the worry tells you. If the challenge seems too difficult, break it up into smaller steps and practice one small step at a time.

Results and Rewards

You'll notice that the more you do it, the easier it gets, so keep practicing. You may need to keep challenging your worry until your body can get used to a new habit or routine. Your body will learn that the situation is not dangerous, and you won't have as many worries about it.

Set appropriate and realistic expectations. Rather than focusing on outside markers of success like awards or compliments, reward yourself for pushing yourself to try, to learn, to grow—that is what leads to a lifetime of happiness and success.

Example: Let's practice using the FEAR plan here. Looks like Michael's alarm is going off.

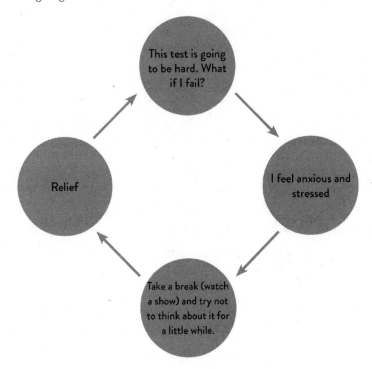

What is he **F**eeling?

He's feeling anxious and stressed.

Expecting bad things to happen?

Yes, he's worrying that he might fail his test.

"Watch out—the bully is trying to get your attention!"

Challenge the thought:

I don't usually fail tests. I'm might make a few mistakes, but that's just because I'm learning something new.

Choose my focus:

What I do have: I understand most of what we've been talking about in class—maybe it won't be too hard.

What I can do: Do the practice sheet my teacher gave and look over my notes. I can see if my friend wants to review together.

Actions that can help:

Do the thing that will most likely lead you to your end goal: Do the worksheet and see if I have any questions. I can ask my friend or my teacher if I don't understand something.

Do the *opposite* of what worry wants you do: Do some work now and then take a break. I'll have something to look forward to instead of something that makes me feel bad because I'm not doing homework.

Results and Rewards:

Plan a break that's fun. Tomorrow I'll feel good that at least I did practice, and I did what I could to prepare.

I (MK) worked with a young woman who struggled with OCD and anxiety during her elementary school years. She became expert at understanding how worries work, where her emotions come from, and what she could do when she felt overwhelmed. Several years later, when she went to college, she returned to give me an update. She said that she noticed many of her peers were really struggling with adjusting to their new lives. They were overwhelmed by the workload, anxious about meeting new people or having to answer questions in class, overdoing partying or other things meant to relieve stress or help to increase self-confidence in the short term. She told me that she had hated having to spend time struggling with anxiety as a young girl and having to go to therapy. But now she could see that the skills she learned were helping her face everyday challenges with much more ease and confidence than those who had never had to learn the skills so early on.

With lots of practice and lots of conversations about awareness, mind-set, and approach, these skills can become new habits for your child. You won't have to plan practices for long, and you won't have to go through charts and worksheets forever. You and your child can just use the language that will remind them what they can do if they are feeling down or worried.

CONVERSATION STARTER You know there are always going to be problems that pop up from time to time and things that you struggle with. But it's still true that even in challenges, you have the ability or the super-power to make things feel better for ourselves, no matter what the situation. You have a superpower. Your mind's ability to think—to create, plan, imagine, see things that you have never seen and even ones that have never existed—is your greatest strength. It also allows you to choose your focus. You can adjust your perspective—choose to focus on what you do have, and what you can do, rather than what you are lacking.

You can choose to focus on your strengths.

You can choose to take action.

You can choose to not give up.

It is your job to keep in mind, in any given moment, that it is not the situation that makes you feel how you feel.

Your thoughts, what you are focusing on, are powerful in influencing your emotional response. Your behaviors are influenced by the combination of both.

And, ultimately your behavioral and emotional response to the situation is creating the outcome, your "reality"—not the situation or the outside world alone.

But your complex and imaginative mind allows you to linger longer on your mistakes, your disappointments, your weaknesses. You can have wealth, but if focused on a loss, you can feel hopeless and deprived. You can be surrounded by friends and family, but if focused on a rejection, can feel alone and unloved.

From just hearing a scary story, or just thinking about a scary outcome, you can initiate a fight-or-flight response. You don't need an actual tiger—you can just think of one. Think of how particularly damaging it is these days, when you are bombarded by stories and reminders of threat online, on television, and in almost every conversation. You can sustain heightened arousal, or "anxiety," all day long, even when you are not in immediate danger.

When you notice anxiety, stress or low mood, ask yourself:

- What have I been feeling?
- What have I been thinking about?
- What have I been doing in response?

Taking a step back to observe yourself gives you space to decide your approach.

This gives you time to create, rather than react.

You can challenge your initial response. You can choose to focus on what you do have, and what you can do. In other words, you can choose your emotional response.

Eventually, for everyday worries or sad feelings, your child won't necessarily need to go through the whole plan; they'll become more efficient at getting "unstuck" by shifting their attention from the bad things to what they can control and want to do next. *What if I don't get invited to her house? I'm loved and am friendly and kind; it's okay if I don't get invited this time, and I can invite her and maybe another friend over to my house the next weekend.* Rather than trying to calculate, prevent, or change things outside of their control, continue to encourage them to focus on and plan for what they can do today to help themself, their family, their friends, or their community. The action doesn't even need to directly counter the challenge—just planning to watch a movie over the weekend with the family can shift focus from something that didn't go the way they wanted to something that they can control.

Key Takeaways

We hope you've noticed that as a parent you are more frequently sharing your values rather than your fears, normalizing both good and bad emotions, modeling and encouraging putting things into perspective, and being a cheerleader more often than a bodyguard or a judge as your child charts their destiny.

We also hope you've adopted a lifestyle of approach for yourself and your family and through your communication and through your actions modeling focus on what you can control, what you do have, and moving quickly toward creating more of what you want.

What am I **F**eeling? Spot the false alarm. The situation is not dangerous—it's just new, difficult, and uncomfortable.

Expecting bad things to happen? Identify your first thought then challenge it. Choose the most accurate and helpful thought. Ask yourself, *Is what I am thinking accurate? Is what I am thinking useful?* If it seems like you are spending too much time thinking about these thoughts, then it's probably not useful. Remember that you've successfully handled other new, uncomfortable, or difficult situations before. Remember how much you do have and how much you can do.

Attitudes and Actions that can help: Choose an action that will get you closer to your goal rather than avoiding the challenge. Remember what you can control: your thoughts and your actions. Do the opposite of what the worry says. If the challenge seems too difficult, break it up into smaller pieces and practice one small step at a time.

Results and Rewards: The more you do something, the easier it gets, so keep practicing. You may need to keep challenging your worry until your body can get used to a new habit or routine. Your body will learn that the situation is not dangerous, and you won't have as many worries about it. Set appropriate and realistic expectations. Rather than focusing on outside markers of success, like awards or compliments, reward yourself for pushing yourself to try, to learn, to grow—that is what opens you up to a lifetime of happiness and success.

CHAPTER 11

Not Just "Survive," Thrive!

My mission in life is not merely to survive, but to thrive; and to do so with some passion, some compassion, some humor, and some style.

—Maya Angelou

The principles and strategies that we've outlined are meant not only to help your child face difficult challenges. When these principles are understood and practiced, they not only make it easier to cope in difficult times but allow us to live a life of passion and purpose, creating a better world for ourself and others, unburdened by fear and self-doubt. Practicing awareness, compassion, and a mind-set of growth, gratitude, and approach in everyday situations, both good and bad, will lead to more positive emotions and experiences overall. We offer you and your child these tools not just to survive—these are tools that will help your child thrive!

Your child has a superpower. They can learn from past mistakes and improve future outcomes. They can choose their focus, adjust their perspective—choose to focus on the strengths, choose to take action, choose to never give up. Now they know not to linger too long on mistakes or disappointments but to learn from them and grow. They can feel overwhelmed or have a fight-or-flight response, but know that they can get back to calm and move forward at any moment—confident that it is not the situation that makes them feel how they feel; rather, it's what they are thinking, what they are focusing on, and old habits of behavior and emotional responding. They know that they can choose their next new response. They can create what comes next.

Creating More of What You Want

We encourage you and your child to use the principles of CBT and the FEAR plan not just as a plan to use in case of emergency, but as a template to work through your thoughts and emotions in daily life. This requires a commitment to the principles not only when problems arise, but regularly—even when good things are happening!

We all tend to focus too much on what we don't have and things that we have little control over. We need to instead practice focusing on what we do have and what we can do. It is hard to focus on the big picture, our strengths, and our goals, especially when things aren't working out. Commit to spend less time stressing over what could go wrong, and more time on doing what you can to make things go right, on what you bring — not in terms of talent or achievements, but in your pure intention of creating and contributing. This will lead to not only less negative emotion, but also more growth and positive experiences, without fear.

Because our body feels so much more comfortable scanning and planning for the worst, it's hard to focus on what we do have, even when things are going well! Have you noticed that when you're feeling happy about something you don't want to think too much about it—for fear you might jinx it? Or do you feel the need to start planning for what might go wrong next, to ensure that things continue to go well? The human mind actually feels more comfortable anticipating danger and planning and worrying. So you and your child need to work to form a habit of thinking about what you can do to create more of what you want and to spend more time on the people, things, and experiences you are grateful for.

But the effort is so worth it. Waking up and, instead of thinking of how you will avoid the problems of the day, thinking of all the things you are grateful for and how you can enjoy and explore your work, family, and friends more. Not only do you feel more at peace, more joyful, and less stressed, but you also put yourself in a position to create and experience more of the things that bring you joy.

Let's imagine you are feeling stressed at work. Your boss has been putting pressure on you about a deadline, and you're feeling like it's going to be almost impossible to get it done on time. You wake up and scan ahead to your day. *How will I finish? Too much to do! Not enough help! Just want a break!* Or you wake up and choose to look around and feel grateful for your home, your family, and the smell of coffee. As you take a deep breath, you remind yourself how much you care about your work. You are imperfect, but you have genuine intent to do everything you can to make the deadline. You'll show up and bring energy and kindness to every room. And right now you will dedicate to making the morning as light as possible as you and your kids get out the door—reminding them, too, that there's nothing they can do wrong today; they are off to learn and grow and share their kindness with their friends and teachers.

Because this may not be an established habit just yet, we offer some activities that can help your child build the habit of scanning for strengths, planning to create joy, and staying in the mind-set of growth and gratitude. Before you begin, think for a minute about what you do that makes you feel excited and full of joy. Hold that feeling for a few more seconds. What do you find yourself doing when you feel the most at peace? What are the things and who are the people you are most grateful for? Now, what is one thing you can do to create more of this feeling in your day today? This is what we will be asking your child to think through and then practice—with your modeling and encouragement—to hold this focus as often and as long as possible.

CONVERSATION STARTER A lot of people think "happy" is just what you are or are not, depending on what's going on in your world that day. Like if something good happens, you feel happy—but if nothing good happens, or something bad happens, you don't. But actually, just like we've been talking about with fears and sad feelings, happiness and good feelings come as much from within us as from what's going on around us. They come from how we're thinking about things and what actions we're choosing, too. So why don't we practice feeling good as often as we can?

When we accomplish a goal, we feel good. When we try something new that we've wanted to try, we feel good. When we do something that helps others, we feel good. We all have different opinions about the things that bring happiness, because happiness has a lot to do with what we as individuals care about—and that is different for each person. For example, some people are happy when they're fishing; other people find fishing to be boring.

So what are your interests? What makes you smile? What makes you feel good? Write these down on a piece of paper, or download the Creating More of What You Want worksheet at http://www.newharbinger.com/46967.

Before you start listing, remember there are some things that make you feel good right away but only for a short time (like eating ice cream or watching a TV show). Then there are things that might not feel great right away but make you feel good for a long time (like working really hard on making your own comic book and then, maybe after a few months, finally finishing it—and getting good at drawing in the process). You might want to list a little of both of those kinds of things.

CONVERSATION STARTER   We often think about all the things we don't want (don't want to have a bad day, don't want homework), and all the things we want more of (more friends, more toys, more holidays). These thoughts make us feel worried, sad, and sometimes even angry.

But if you can pause and focus on the things you already have, the bad things become like little obstacles that you might notice but not need to give much time and energy to. When you're having a tough day, it helps to think of the things you're grateful for. When we focus on the things we're grateful for, we feel good. And when we feel good, we put more energy and joy into everything we do, which then makes our whole day better. Let's try to make our days brighter as often as possible. Take a few minutes to list the things that you are grateful for.

You can use the I Am Grateful For... form (available for download at http://www.newharbinger.com/46967), or design your own form, or you can be start a gratitude journal in a little notebook or on your computer or phone. Every day you can record the things you are grateful for. It's a great way to start choosing what to focus on and what to fill your day with.

It's okay to repeat the same things on different days—that just means you're really lucky to have that great thing or person in your life! Eventually, you can try to think of new things to list or focus on a different aspect of that person or thing.

Make it a habit to write down what you are grateful for daily (try first thing in the morning or right before bed). It just takes a couple of minutes. Don't think of it as a chore—consider it a time when you get to think about good stuff and feel good.

Here are some other prompts:

- Things or people who make me laugh

- Three nice things that happened today

- The people who love me

- My environment

- Experiences (interesting, fun, or learning adventures that I've had)

- Tastes and smells (yummy foods or items that always smell nice)

- Times people have been kind to me

- Things that I am proud of

- People or things that make my life easier or nicer

- People who help me, such as teachers, coaches, doctors, firefighters, and so on

- The everyday things that I might forget about (the car, bus, train, or plane that takes me where I need to go; grocery stores that have my favorite foods; traffic lights so people don't get stuck at corners; sports team that I like to watch and cheer for; my brain, for making me so smart!)

Healthy Body = Healthy Mind

There are obvious benefits of healthy diet and exercise for our physical well-being. Perhaps less obvious, but absolutely real, are the significant benefits of healthy diet and exercise for mental health. Aerobic exercise, including jogging, swimming, cycling, walking, and dancing, has been shown to reduce feelings of anxiety and depression (Peluso & Guerra de Andrade, 2005), as well as improve sleep, energy, and motivation, and reduce our natural stress response (fight-or-flight), which means we feel less anxious and stressed in general. Try to keep your child on a routine that includes some type of exercise and/or spending time outdoors—aim for at least an hour per day, weather permitting (and indoors, there's always dancing and active games).

We find that establishing a routine works better than keeping a to-do list for reaching healthy lifestyle goals. A routine is something you don't have to think about each day—it's more of a plan to keep for most days/most weeks. With a routine, you wake up around the same time weekday mornings and go to bed around the same time on weeknights, with a slightly different but similar sleep routine on weekends. Homework is at a certain part of the day on weeknights and on weekends. Meals are usually around the same time on weeknights. When something is routine, it becomes habit, so it's less likely we'll have trouble getting started. Establishing a routine for something difficult or uncomfortable (like doing homework or going to a lesson or sports practice) is usually the hardest part. As soon as our alarm system scans something uncomfortable coming, it gives us the signal to escape. With a routine, the alarm goes off less, because by doing something every day or most days at about the same time, our body learns that it's not dangerous, so it sends our mind the message that all is okay. We spend less time struggling with uncertainty about what's next and what's the best way to spend this hour, and it makes it easier to get through that getting-started period and do the things we know are healthy but aren't always the most fun or immediately gratifying. Routines also provide the stability and structure that are reassuring to children and really important for well-being. As with every aspect of this resilience recipe, keep in mind that routines will be imperfect, life will get in the way, and you and your child will need to make adjustments and handle interruptions to the routine, more often than not. But you'll know that your child can always go back to the routine and back to that healthy lifestyle.

There are similarly obvious benefits to social interaction. You'll see mood and flexibility improve with more time with friends and family. One of the most difficult challenges of the COVID-19 pandemic has been the way it cut us off from the social interaction we were used to. Our brains and bodies don't do well in isolation. The social isolation period has been difficult for all of us, but particularly for children and adolescents, who are in the midst of developing their social identities and autonomy. We've seen the isolation lead to withdrawal, irritability, regression, and even self-destructive behaviors. Young brains crave social connectedness, and the necessary safety precautions have gotten in the way of that. Until we enter a new normal—whatever that may be—it's important to keep encouraging different ways to interact and connect with people of their own age and of other ages.

Again, having a routine where socialization is just part of daily life is ideal. Onsite, in-person school provides some of this in a structured way that is very helpful for those children who are more shy or still developing social skills and confidence. Other types of structured social connection can come from structured camps, local theater, sports, music, art classes, or helping in a community effort. Unstructured social time—playing outside with friends, calling grandparents, even writing emails or thank-you cards, all are extremely valuable for improving overall well-being. You'll see mood and flexibility improve with more time with friends and family. Don't forget to include some time with you doing unstructured things together, rather than trying to accomplish or improve something. You might try reading the same book series, playing a video game together, or a sport your child loves to play (even if you may not really enjoy it), watching a show series together (perhaps while on video call with kids who are living outside of your home).

Every study on happiness and resilience will tell you that what really keeps us healthy and happy is the amount of time we spend with the people we love. So make your routine include lots of time with friends and family.

Key Takeaways

When these principles are understood and practiced, they not only make it easier to cope in difficult times, but also allow us to live a life of passion and purpose, creating a better world for ourselves and others, unburdened by fear and self-doubt.

We encourage you and your child to use the principles of CBT and the FEAR plan as a template to work through your thoughts and emotions in daily life, as opposed to a plan to use just in case of emergency. This requires a commitment to the principles not only when problems arise, but on a regular basis—even when good things are happening!

Commit to making it your job to "shrink" the time spent on what could go wrong and expanding the amount of time spent on what you can do to make go right. Focus on what you bring—not in terms of talent or achievements, but in your pure intention of creating and contributing. This will lead to not only less negative emotion, but also more growth and positive experiences—without fear.

What do you find yourself doing when you feel the most at peace? What are the things and who are the people you are most grateful for? Now, what is one thing you can do to create more of this feeling in your day today?

If you can pause and focus on the things you already have, the bad things become like little obstacles that you might notice but not need to give much time and energy to. When you're having a tough day, it helps to think of the things you're grateful for. When we focus on the things we're grateful for, we feel good. And when we feel good, we put more energy and joy in everything we do which then makes our whole day better.

Try to keep your child on a routine that includes some type of exercise and/or spending time outdoors—shoot for at least an hour per day.

Make a plan and create a routine that will make it most likely that you can stick with the plan. Think first of things that are enjoyable and meaningful.

CHAPTER 12

Parenting in the Age of Anxiety

Pain is inevitable, suffering is optional...we have bigger houses, but smaller families. More conveniences, but less time. We have knowledge, but less judgment; more experts, but more problems; more medicines but less health.

—Dalai Lama

Today, more than triple the number of children have an anxiety disorder and/or depression than did just ten years ago. In a 2020 *Atlantic* article investigating this rise in mental health problems in children and teens in the US, author Kate Julien writes, "To my surprise, as I began interviewing experts [and] parents...the people I spoke with emphasized...how we might head off more [emotional disorders] at the pass. The when: childhood.... The how: treatment of anxiety..."

We agree that, in addition to helping our children develop self-awareness and bring choice into their emotional and behavioral responses in general, teaching them how to manage anxiety is critical to helping them build resilience and confidence to face future challenges. Anxiety is a sneaky enemy because it hides within what seems, in the moment, to be our own good planning. But we are navigating uncharted waters in unprecedented times. How do we prepare our children for what we have no experience with ourselves? While we don't have the answers to the problems that exist, nor can we predict all of the challenges that will arise in our children's future, here we provide some suggestions for what we as parents can do to help them feel confident in themselves and their world. We must guide our children toward positive and effective ways to manage negative emotions and reduce stress, otherwise many will develop negative thinking styles that can lead to a lifetime of struggles with anxiety and depression, and many will choose destructive behaviors to find relief. We can change the trajectory of mental health suffering in our children and future generations by changing our approach to new challenges.

The Overwhelm: Mass Shootings, Social Injustices, Climate Change, and Global Pandemic

Children of the twenty-first century are subjected to a constant stream of news of many crises—local, national, and global. They hear of many mass shootings—particularly, and most frighteningly for children and parents, in schools. They hear of political divisions, civil unrest, race- and gender-related violence, and the ongoing struggles in the fight against discrimination based on race, gender, and sexuality. Our children have been hearing and learning about climate change and its impact on the future of our planet their whole lives. We knew it would be among the greatest challenges in our lifetime, and most certainly of theirs. Just when we began acknowledging that climate change demanded our immediate attention, the COVID-19 pandemic hit. The pandemic brought a new immediacy to how the actions of others affect our own personal health and freedom—and vice versa—in a way that climate change had not yet done. We won't know for some time the full impact of the COVID-19 pandemic on the social-emotional development of youth, but it will likely be significant. What these crises all have in common is that they confront us with forces beyond our control that make us vulnerable and threaten our lives and our futures.

Without immediate solutions, there is uncertainty—and as we've discussed, whenever there is uncertainty, our built-in alarm goes off. Without control, without certainty, there is a natural tendency to feel anxious. During the pandemic all of us, individually and collectively, have experienced anxiety, and many even experienced a trauma. Those of us who are vulnerable to anxiety have struggled even more with managing the frequent and intense alarms. From our perspective as anxiety researchers, it seems certain that the experience of hearing and witnessing stories of death and disease daily reinforces beliefs that the world is dangerous—that we are not safe, that we do not have any control over our future—and this would predictably lead to more anxiety for all of us (see the worry cycle figure, "What if I get sick?").

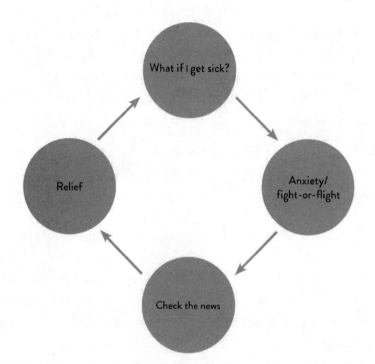

What can we do to help our children with crises like these? Let's go back to the principles. In every situation, regardless of the circumstance, our response to the situation is made up of our chosen interpretation of the situation (thoughts), which brings about emotions and a set of actions (behaviors). While we may not be able to immediately influence the situation, we can immediately take charge of our thoughts and behaviors and influence our emotional experience. When outside forces are moving in a way that seem uncontrollable, the first thing we can do is to acknowledge that while there are many things outside of our control, there are also things within our control that we can focus on. For example,

- I can't control someone else wearing or not wearing a mask, but I can choose to wear a mask myself.

- While I can't control whether the energy company will get the lights working again today, I can control staying focused on being grateful that my family is safe at home.

- While I can't make others less racist, I know I can make choices that support those who are discriminated against, remove support from people and policies that maintain discrimination, and live and act under the principle that I will treat others as I wish to be treated.

We can also choose to take more action, but we must understand that it is only the action we can control, not a particular outcome. When you take this approach and model it, using your actions and words, your child will learn how to handle uncertainty and challenge—knowledge that reduces the feeling of lack of control and increases confidence in their own ability to manage a challenge. This part is critical.

The future is inherently uncertain. Every day we wake up not knowing what the day holds. When our mind finds uncertainty, instead of outlining *all* of the possibilities, it attends to the negative possibilities. And when we start to focus on these possible negative outcomes, we feel anxious—more anxious than the circumstances of the day, or our future, necessarily calls for. But this is how our mind works—it scans for danger to try to keep us safe. It's not helpful, though, when we are safe and anticipating danger. It's not particularly helpful even when there is some danger—our attention would be better used focusing on problem solving, not fighting, fleeing, or freezing.

Our power over this initial instinct, and over our overall experience, lies not in trying to control the outcome, but in knowing that we can manage any situation. We don't need certainty of the future because we know no matter what, we can manage it—we can survive, we can problem solve, we can find the best way to get the best outcome possible. Certainty lies within us. The messages to your child: "While there are many things outside of our control, there are also things within our control that we can focus on," and "You don't know what's going to happen, but you do know you'll make it turn out as well as possible."

Smartphones and Social Media

Many have hypothesized—and some have concluded—that smartphones and social media are to blame for the sharp increase in depression and anxiety in young people in the last decade. While there are many reasons that make intuitive sense to believe that this is the primary driver, and there are studies that have documented serious negative effects (more on this shortly), there are many studies that have found little to no effect of screen time on adolescent well-being. Many teens and tweens report feeling less depressed and lonely as a result of having social media and text messaging.

Mobile communication technology itself is not a crisis—it is a step forward in human history, and its benefits to our lives are innumerable. However, daily life in the US and around the world has been forever altered—everything from our daily routines to our values and relationships. With such a seismic change in lifestyle and society more generally, it's understandable that new problems will arise and adjustments must be made. Unfortunately, the technology came before our understanding of its influence on our behaviors. Before we knew enough to establish healthy rules and routines, we were given 24/7 access to news, information, media, and an expanding social network that now includes distant relatives, old friends, neighbors, and strangers from around the world.

According to the Pew Internet & American Life Project, today about 95 percent of teens in the US have or have access to a smartphone or mobile device—a 22 percent increase from 2015. Smartphone ownership is nearly universal, with few differences across genders, ethnicities and races, and socioeconomic backgrounds. On average, teens are online almost nine hours per day, not including time for homework. Daily use of computers for homework has doubled. This number will undoubtedly increase, as it already has since the advent of the pandemic. Psychologist Jean Twenge found that teens who spend three hours per day or more on an electronic device are 35 percent more likely and those who spend five hours or more are 71 percent more likely to have a risk for suicide than those who spend less than one hour (Twenge et al., 2017). Other data from the United States and the United Kingdom show that the incidence of body dysmorphia and eating disorders has risen by approximately 30 percent among late adolescent-age girls since the advent of social media (see, for example, Smink, van Hoeken, & Hoek, 2012).

In the face of this, most parents feel at a loss—should we limit smartphones or other screens for our kids? But how, when even schools are requiring technology for homework and, as we've seen during the pandemic, video-teleconferencing? We are in a situation where it may not be feasible to reduce the number of hours our children spend on an electric device.

While we can't say definitively what's the "right" amount of time to spend on a screen per day or whether screen time increases anxiety, depression, eating disorders, or suicide, we recommend bolstering your children's "electronic intelligence" to help them have a healthy relationship with screens and social media.

We can return to the principles we offer in this book to help us find ways to minimize the negative impact of social media and screen time on our children's physical, social, and emotional well-being.

Have you noticed that it's hard to stop checking your phone, even when you know you should? Our phones, tablets, and other screens are hard to stay away from not just because they are useful tools for communication and task completion. They are also very powerful reinforcers—through both positive and negative reinforcement—of the behavior of checking. In other words, we keep checking them because it feels very rewarding (positive reinforcement) or relieving (negative reinforcement) every time we check our news feed, social media, and/or messages. Every time we get a "like" or a compliment, or see something funny, or learn something new, we feel good—this is positive reinforcement—and we will be more likely to seek this out, especially when we are feeling stressed, bored, or down. Every time we get a "like" we are also reassured that we are liked and included, and/or that we are not missing out on important information (be it news or gossip), as well as the relief we get from a brief escape from difficult tasks. These are all powerful negative reinforcers. Comparing your opinions and abilities against others, or social comparison (such as checking someone else's profile or feed; Festinger, 1954) is a check too—a check of how you are doing relative to someone else. We have all experienced how negative and emotionally draining social comparison can feel. Sometimes it can have a positive consequence, like learning something new, motivating change, or gaining pride in our own abilities or characteristics. But our brains are primed to scan for danger, so more often than not, comparing ourselves with others on characteristics such as appearance, popularity, and success becomes a negative exercise.

Our alarms will sound, telling us to work hard to prevent or fix any problems so we don't feel we're not doing as well as others. In the case of social media, a quick fix can be as simple as using a filter before posting a photo, or posting comments that exude qualities we think others value, or even planning an event to show how well we're doing. These fixes actually bring relief but then reinforce checking again! Our brain anticipates danger (such as, rejection or failure) and seeks relief through fixing or checking. Our smartphone is a 24/7 source of worry that lives in our pocket! We find ourselves checking our phones even when we know it's not the right time, because we feel good when we do. And over time, it feels like if we don't check, the opposite might happen—we will discover that we are not liked, or we have been left out, or we missed out on important information, or that we are inferior or unsuccessful, so we *must check*. Just like all behaviors that come from a worry cycle, if we do enough checking and fixing, they become interfering (see the worry cycle figure, "What if they don't like me?").

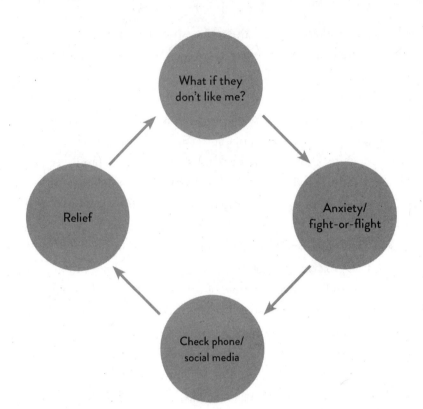

Both adults and children struggle to free themselves from this worry cycle. The fear of social rejection is one of our strongest fear instincts, and it takes effort and practice to counter it and do the opposite. You might know from your own experience how hard it is to ignore social judgment, to not seek validation from others, to know your own self-worth, or to not need to evaluate where you are relative to others. We adults struggle with this, so certainly children—who have not had time to practice and develop social skills and understanding or to develop confidence in their own self-worth—struggle even more. It is important to help them identify this cycle so they can keep themselves from getting into a cycle of worry and checking that becomes interfering and generates more anxiety and low self-esteem. We want to communicate that as much as checking is a natural instinct to protect from rejection, it's a worry cycle (awareness), and we must break it by remembering what we do have (people who love and value us; mind-set) and what we can do (plan to give love, not check love). So we let the phone buzz, or we sit in a different room (it is uncomfortable, but not dangerous; approach) while we are trying to stay present with someone or something else.

The Value of Routines

In addition to helping our kids identify and challenge the worry cycle, it is also important to create healthy routines around social media and screen access. Routines often save us when we are fighting off powerful instincts, such as relief-seeking. We can develop routines that make it harder to fall into the trap of the opportunity to "check" or "fix" or "protect" around the clock. Yes, it is helpful to be aware of the worry cycle, and to plan actions to guide you as you actively fight the urge to check. But routines are what really help us stick to our goals with less struggle. They help us so we don't fall into the trap in the first place. You wake up, take a shower, have breakfast, and go to work, not because those are necessarily the things you'd choose to do every day, but because they're in line with your long-term goals and values, and you've created a routine to make it less of a struggle. Routines help our kids, too—sitting down to do homework at the same time every day can be less of a struggle than sitting down to do a mass of homework once every few days (there's a reason why it's so hard to get back into school after a holiday break).

Routines don't feel like punishment, so there is also less of a power struggle. For instance, if you've made a routine of video games only on the weekends, it's less of a power struggle than trying to limit video games on weeknights. Many children are using their phones in the hours before bedtime, despite the American Academy of Pediatrics recommendation that children not sleep with their devices in their bedrooms and stop using screen media at least an hour before bedtime. About 30 percent of teens take their phones to bed with them. One practice to change these habits is to create a home hub away from the bedrooms for charging phones overnight, and establish a family routine of putting the phones to charge when it's time for bed. For older children who may be up later, there could be a routine of charging in a closed box charger rather than on their bedside table when they get into bed, and putting a book on the bedside table to read when they are trying to get to sleep instead of watching a show or scrolling through their Instagram. We recommend starting as early as possible to create healthy routines for phones and screens that work best for your family; it's easier to start when children are younger and still depending on you to guide their day's structure.

Similarly, we recommend, for both kids and parents, that you keep the routine of checking news and news-related social media to only once or twice per day—perhaps once after breakfast and once after dinner. You won't miss anything *and* you'll be more present and relaxed throughout the day. When our brain detects uncertainty on a local level, because it is designed to protect us—to seek information that can keep us safe—there's always a really strong pull to access news. The irony is that the more you seek information, the more anxious you tend to feel, sending your brain the message that you *are* in danger. You end up actually repeating the worry in your mind, which increases your anxiety, which then leads you to want to check the news again! Before long, you are stuck in a worry cycle in which *you are not really seeking information anymore; rather, you are seeking reassurance*—anything that might provide some relief—either through escape or through reassuring news, and this includes social media.

Help Them Bridge the Gap

Our children are *native users* of mobile technology (those of us who were already adults when smartphones and social media were invented are considered *immigrant users*) and, in a way, further along than the immigrants in understanding the "new normal" in social relationships. But they may have missed out on some learning about interpersonal communication, building relationships, and managing social rejection that, in the absence of mobile technology, occurs more organically and on a smaller scale. Children and adolescents are still developing their identity, their understanding of who they are in the world. This is why we urge parents to wait as long as possible to give their children their own smartphones. The delay gives them more opportunity to develop their own identity and try out different approaches on a small, personal scale where they can adjust and grow at their own pace. The social network can be too quick to judge, and too many influences and opinions appear at once, making it difficult to learn incrementally. Children and teens lack the life experience to bring balance to positive and negative experiences, so rejection becomes even harder to take, and the fear of rejection harder to ignore. We must help them bridge this gap, because they can easily fall into a cycle of worry. If they join a social platform or group chat before they've developed skills to manage it, they may quickly experience rejection in a larger social world. The anonymity of the internet allows people to act out cruelty more easily, so social rejection can be more intense than it would typically be in face-to-face interactions.

We recommend having conversations early and often about meaningful relationships and friendships, and the differences between a good friend, an acquaintance, and a stranger—and how to apply this understanding to online friendships. The main points:

- We can't control what other people do, but we can control what we choose to do (e.g., giving love rather than checking love) and who we choose to be with.

- Expect that people will come in and out of your life; the ones who stay in longest are the ones who have proven themselves to be good friends.

- Stay focused on the things that you can control, what you do have, and the people you are grateful for.

- Avoid oversharing personal information, and become more of an observer or evaluator of content rather than a consumer.

A Culture of Perfectionism: Fear of Failure

Remember, our beliefs are shaped by our learning history, our biological predispositions, and our culture. Our beliefs about success and happiness are no different. How would you define success? Where did that definition come from? What factors that can lead to success are in your control? Do they guarantee success? We need to be very aware of our beliefs about success and happiness, as these drive many of our day-to-day thoughts and actions, and therefore what we communicate to our kids.

One particularly dominant philosophy has been the fabric of US culture since the country's founding: if you work hard, you can succeed. Our culture values perfection, and it purports that perfection is achievable, if you work hard enough. It's drilled into us that our homes should be Instagrammable, our bodies should be magazine cover ready, our travels luxurious, and our relationships made for fairy tales. We inadvertently (or purposefully) teach our kids in school and at home, through television shows, movies, and books, that they can achieve better grades, have more success in sports, look more attractive, have more friends, get into a "good" college, which will set them up for a "good" job and a nicer house and fancier car, if they just work hard enough—harder than everyone else (see Curran & Hill, 2017).

Our kids are spending more time and more years in school than in any previous generation. There's increased focus on and valuation of grades and athletics, not necessarily for the fun and exhilaration of pursuit and sport, but to achieve specific external outcomes such as scholarships and accolades. As we have noted, there is no one factor creating increased anxiety and depression in our children, and certainly we do not have data to show any causal links for any specific factor(s), but an increased focus on school academic and athletic performance outcomes, with a system that claims to guarantee outcomes if one puts in enough effort, may be contributing.

There is no disputing the advantages of a democracy where citizens have the freedom to pursue happiness, and of a culture that promotes grit, determination, and drive. However, there are dangers to the promotion of effort, in and of itself, as the channel to success. Success as a function of effort alone would also mean that if you haven't succeeded (say, didn't get the job you wanted, or didn't get into your first-choice university), you didn't work hard enough. This can become a source of guilt, shame, hopelessness, and self-loathing.

Those who have faced discrimination or socioeconomic disadvantage, or seen privilege accorded to others, will tell you that hard work isn't the only factor in academic or career achievement in this or any other country. It's unnecessary to point out the countless very hard-working individuals—young and old, rich and poor, male and female—who for various reasons may never achieve the external metrics of success as our society define them.

Not only is the premise of effort = success a fallacy, but it implies that anything other than perfection indicates some failing on the individual's part—a lack of discipline, effort, perseverance, hustle, or grit. These are qualities we have come to revere, so if these are what we lack, we feel guilt, shame, and self-loathing. Further, defining success using metrics such as grades, college rank, job title, size of house or type of car leaves our self-worth in the hands of too many outside factors—things beyond our control. Worse, defining personal success by things outside oneself undervalues the self.

Our goal is to encourage kids to be resilient, to pursue and grow, all while free from the burden of fear. If we try to motivate or encourage them to pursue success by using threats or scare stories of failure, their efforts to succeed will be born of fighting or fleeing the specter of failure. This means they'll experience anxiety throughout, and they'll build a new learning that they are incapable of tolerating failure (or any obstacle or difficulty)—precisely the opposite of learning resilience.

Especially if you see your child struggling with anxiety or stress, or seeming to shy away from challenge, or withdrawing from pursuits that could put them at risk of rejection or failure, or even becoming more irritable and obstinate in the face of challenges, it may be that too many threats of failure or stories that hard work equals success have not motivated them, but rather incited a fight-or-flight response (see the worry cycle figure What if I Fail?).

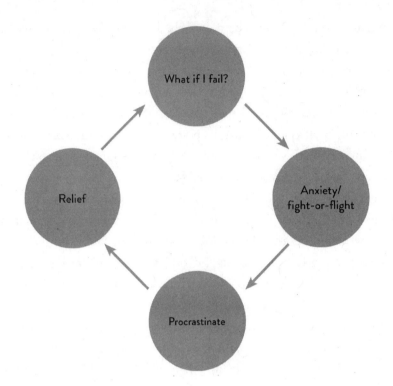

We recommend reminding your child to focus on what they do have and what they can do: develop and practice the process (for example, finishing homework at the same time each day before checking their phone) that will ultimately lead to success rather than focusing on the outcome of their performance (for example, being selected for a scholarship), which they can't control. We encourage them to be more general, rather than specific, in thinking about their expectations for the future ("I will work to help those who are suffering" versus "I will graduate from UVA medical school"). We want them to be clear on the big-picture importance of things ("I'm practicing and getting better each day"), rather than getting caught up in the specific, sometimes man-made or self-made pressures ("I won the match"). Most important, we want them to know that their value, their worth, is not in question. They were born worthy, and nothing can take that away. No man-made rules about what is "smart" or what is "attractive" or what is "success" can change that they are inherently worthy of love, respect, and appreciation.

You may think, *Of course they know I love and value them; that goes without saying!* but you may not want to let it go too long without saying, or while modeling the opposite beliefs too often. They are looking to us first to know if they are valued and appreciated for who they are. Even when they are arguing with us, they are seeking our approval and acceptance. Your child is born with the natural instinct to pursue, grow, and love. This natural instinct will lead to a lifetime of joy and, in the process, many successes. Why not celebrate with them? The message to your child: "I know you are smart—I don't need this test to tell me." "You are learning more every day; it will seem easier after some more practice." "You don't know how the test will go, but you do know you'll never fail because you'll never stop trying."

We are *not* promoting mediocrity or claiming that we do not have any control over our fate and are products of our circumstances—in fact, quite the opposite. We are promoting helping our children reach their fullest potential despite any circumstance. We argue that in order for anyone to be in a position to achieve their highest aspirations, to pursue greatness and push to the fullest extent of their potential, they first must not be burdened by fear of failure.

A Growth Mindset

Stanford psychologist Dr. Carol Dweck has studied and written about success and resilience for decades. Dweck's research on performance has really informed our work with anxiety and perfectionism. Dweck found that one key to reducing stress and improving performance was to have a *growth mindset*—that is, to think *not yet: I haven't gotten there yet, but with practice I will get there*—as opposed to a fixed mindset (*I'm not that smart; I'm bad at math*), the fixed state in which you are stuck and things will never change.

When children and teens struggle with worries about failure or underperforming, we need to help them challenge their anxious thoughts by remembering to focus on process, not outcome. We want them to measure themselves not by the outcome of their performance, which they can't control, but on the process that will ultimately lead to success. We too make the mistakes of communicating a fixed mindset—"You're not a math person" or "Why are you so lazy?" rather than "You just didn't get it yet" or "It's hard, but doing a little will make the next part seem easier—the more you do, the easier it will get." Too often, we ask outcome-based questions after the fact:

"How'd the test go?"

"Are you finished with the book report?"

"Did you make it to the finals?"

Questions about process are asked *before* the event takes place, to show where your values lie:

"How did planning or training go?"

"Did you feel like you learned what this unit was about? If not, what would you want to do to feel more comfortable with the content?"

"Is there anything you'd like to keep doing or something you'd do differently?"

"Have you been able to keep the importance of this one event/test/ outcome in perspective?"

We want children to focus on the learning and the fun of new information, sharing opinions and conversation with others who are informed, and exploring how to solve problems:

"What was the story about? What did you think of that?"

"Here's why I've always thought that Rosa Parks was such an important figure in history."

"Right, that's sort of why we're so worried about climate change—do you think we're ever going to be able to reverse the damage?"

Encourage them through conversation to think about the big picture, not their semester or college goals. What are their dreams? What kind of skills will they need to pursue these dreams? Probably not all A's, but persistence, problem solving, creativity, teamwork, and purpose. Use these words more often when communicating what you think is important and what leads to success.

We must give our kids permission to fail. We are not all-knowing. We do not have the answers or the ability to prevent loss and grief. They will face many challenges—new and different from the ones we have faced—so our solutions may not apply. Rather than taking the wheel, we must let them drive, learn how to be prepared, stay alert, but also be able to enjoy the wind in their hair.

A Bright Future

Instead of being afraid of these new and ongoing challenges, we must stay aware and compassionate. Instead of falling prey to fear and anxiety, we should stay focused on what we do have and what we can do.

There is much to feel good and hopeful about our children's future. The US child population is more diverse than ever before. There are more youth-led efforts to demand action than there were in decades prior. While we all know Greta and Malala, there are thousands of others working tirelessly around the world for causes including combating climate change and working for racial and gender equality, LGBTQ rights, and social change.

It Takes Two to Talk

In Kate Julien's *Atlantic* article, she describes the vicious cycle that today's parents have experienced, in which parental stress leads to child stress, which leads to more parental stress, which has led to "an epidemic of anxiety at all ages." As a parent of a Gen Z or iGen child, I (MK) have found myself stuck in this vicious cycle as well.

When my son was a toddler he was not on track with developing language as would be expected for his age. A researcher by nature, I immediately started doing hours of research about language delays and language development. We got an evaluation and started working with our intermediary unit on speech and language classes.

In my research, I found an evidence-based manual for parents to help their children with language delays: "It Takes

Two to Talk," by Elaine Weitzman. In the first few pages—
even just in its title—it sparked an "aha!" moment for me.
My son had great eye contact, friendly and appropriate affect,
strong nonverbal communication, and several words—just
fewer than the lower cutoff of normal range. This wasn't a
developmental delay. He could learn and speak words—but
he needed someone to communicate with him. Not talk *to*
him, like when reading words from a book, but talk *with*
him—asking him questions, explaining what was going on,
laughing at things that were funny…of course! That's how our
brains learn language!

I know this must sound obvious to you as you read this,
but these truths had slipped under my radar. For all the things
I thought I was doing right—from baby gates to nursing to
sleep training—my son wasn't having enough conversations
throughout his day.

I was a working mother of two under age four. I worked as
a clinical psychologist and researcher at a medical school that
was a teaching hospital and research powerhouse. I was doing
my research and teaching during the day, seeing patients
during the after-school/after-work hours, and writing grants
late at night and on weekends. My husband was an executive
at a tech company that needed him to be available at a
moment's notice to travel at least once or twice per week. This
meant we were often working late and always running. So late
that daycares didn't work for us. We had au pairs because they
had more flexible hours than daycare, and my husband and
I could make it work. The years my son was developing
language, we had an Indian au pair. She was warm and loving,
but her English was not strong. She spent hours with my
son—using language that no one else in the house was using
(I am a native Bengali speaker, my husband a native Hindi
speaker, so we speak English at home, and she spoke Punjabi).

I was with my son mornings and bedtimes and weekends, but always rushed so I could get everything in. In the evenings, I would quickly give him a bath, read a book with some pointing at pictures and character voices, and then put him down to sleep so I could start that same routine again with my daughter before it got too late. When I was with him in the morning, it was another rush to get everyone ready and fed, lunches packed, and run out the door. The weekends were busy with cooking, cleaning, birthday parties and play-dates, time with family and friends, and trying to maintain date night. I was stressed, but being a cognitive behavioral therapist, I stayed positive and energized by reminding myself that I was tired, but I was grateful to be able to do everything I loved. I was your typical supermom who could do it all. Or could I?

When I had the "aha!" moment, I knew things had to change. I had to make more time to be with my son when he was alert and awake. I took two mornings a week off and worked later on those days. I stopped using my weekends to write. My grant writing certainly suffered, and I published less, but I would have made that choice a million times over. I was lucky that my boss, mentor, and colleague, Dr. Martin Franklin (whom I will still thank to this day) helped me make the adjustments to my schedule without hurting my position. I know not all parents have that kind of support.

I spent the mornings playing with my son, laughing and hugging—and we talked! It was just the two of us, and I made sure my mind was only on him. On the weekends, I made sure to spend time with my kids being more present and engaged—doing less for myself and others. Within about six months he was multiplying the number of words he used, and just one year later he was back on target for language ability in his age range. Today, he is advanced in his reading, writing, and public speaking abilities and, more important, is one of the most enjoyable conversationalists I know.

I bring this story up because for me it was a concrete and clear demonstration of the inherent impossibilities and hypocrisies of modern life—and highlights some of the many reasons we parents are stressed. While there are many benefits and advantages of a two-working-parent household, there are also many challenges and disadvantages for families. Grandparents are working later in life or living independently, making their support less available. The current rate of divorce in the US is between 40 and 50 percent of marriages. Divorce has far-reaching impacts on adults' well-being, with increased stress on individual finances, time, and responsibilities. There is a cultural acceptance of work-related travel and 24/7 availability. We wear our lack of sleep and long work hours as a badge of honor. But the "supermom" moniker is not a compliment—it is yet another impossible expectation set on mothers.

This whole episode also reminded me of a fundamental truth: that what children need to develop their brains is time communicating with their parent(s) and/or caregiver(s). This is also what they need to develop their character and their confidence. Parent-child communication is the foundation on which a child develops other social relationships. It builds the foundation for a child's understanding of themselves and others. It takes two to communicate because it involves giving and receiving ideas. It involves talking and listening, time and attention, understanding and respect. But for many reasons, including some of the ones discussed already, it is becoming harder and harder for parents and children to communicate.

Face-to-face time has actually increased since the 1950s. There is research that suggests parents are more involved in their children's lives and for longer—leading to new terms like "helicopter parenting" and "tiger mom." But it may be that the type of engagement has changed as well. According to a study on changes in parent-child relationships in the last thirty years, we are more likely to be monitoring and managing our children's activities and also more likely to be accessible to be able to meet a child's needs, but less engaged in direct, one-on-one interaction—reportedly no more than one hour per day of direct interaction (Montemayor, 1982).

Until systems and societal norms and values shift, sacrifices will have to be made—something will have to give. In my case, these included sacrificing self-care, financial and career aspirations, family and social relationships, volunteerism, and sleep. All of us are making tough choices at every turn. We are all finding ways to deal with these obstacles in various ways, but each solution has its own challenges—and hence, the vicious cycle.

Again, I'm not recommending my path, rather offering it as an example that we're all struggling to make it work, with more or less success from one day to the next. But to support development of new skills, it does take conversation and practice. Your child needs guidance, and better they get it from you than from media influencers, their social network, or less informed peers. Throughout this book we have offered conversation starters to help start those conversations that we hope will get you there effectively and efficiently.

It has been a privilege to share our work with you. We have worked for decades with children and families to develop and evaluate techniques that help build confidence and resilience. All of this work was done with the intention of one day sharing with you what we have learned. We are thrilled to be able to now hand these tools over to you. We hope that we've done so in a way that is practical and clear so that you can use them at home.

We reiterate that this is a long-term strategy, not a quick fix. The skills can become habit and build confidence, but only with repetition and continuing approach of new and more difficult challenges as they grow—and certainly failures, loss, and heartache from time to time. Writing down thoughts, mapping out a worry cycle, and working through the FEAR plan can guide the process of what to do next. If you are part of the cycle (that is, providing fixes, safety nets, or removing barriers for your child), this is the part you can control. Know that a little discomfort today can spare you and your child years of anxiety and stress. You can also control creating a healthy lifestyle, encouraging new and varied activities, including social connectedness and exercise and relaxation, meditation or mindfulness, and disconnecting from phones and news as part of a routine. There will be days that you can do some of this, all of this, and none of this, but be compassionate with yourself and know that your intention to give and love is enough, and get back to the plan of healthy lifestyle again.

Key Takeaways

- Fear of uncertainty: Our power over this initial instinct, and over our overall experience, lies not in knowing or controlling the outcome, but knowing that we can manage it. Certainty lies within us.

- Fear of social rejection: Our brains anticipate danger (such as rejection or failure) and seek relief through fixing or checking. Our phone is a 24/7 source of worry that lives in our pocket! Checking is a natural instinct to protect us from rejection, but it's a worry cycle (awareness) and we must break it by remembering what we do have (people who love and value us; mind-set), what we can do (plan to give love, not check love) and letting the phone buzz or ding or sit in a different room (it is uncomfortable, but not dangerous; approach) while we are trying to stay present with someone or something else.

- Fear of failure:
  - We can't control the outcome, but we can control the process.
  - Good process is what leads to success, not good grades.
  - Remember Carol Dweck—growth mind-set—"You just didn't get there yet. Not yet."
  - Focus on learning and fun (build intrinsic motivation).
  - Flexibility is part of good process.
  - What are their dreams? What kind of skills will they need to pursue these dreams? Probably not all A's, but persistence, problem solving, creativity, teamwork, purpose.

- This is a long-term strategy, not a quick fix. The skills can become habit and build confidence, but only with repetition and continuing approach of new and more difficult challenges as children grow—and certainly failures, loss, and heartache from time to time.

- Writing down thoughts, mapping out a worry cycle, and working through the FEAR plan can guide the process of what to do next.

- If you are part of the cycle (for example, providing fixes, safety nets, or removing barriers), this is the part you can control. Know that a little discomfort today can spare you years of anxiety and stress.

- You can also control creating a healthy lifestyle, encouraging new and varied activities, including social connectedness and exercise and relaxation, meditation or mindfulness, and disconnecting from phones and news as part of a routine.

The FEAR Plan

What am I *Feeling*?

- Identify physiological symptoms: Is it a fight-or-flight false alarm?

- Try some deep breathing.

Expecting bad things to happen?

- Pay attention to thoughts and what "might happen."

- Just because you've thought it doesn't mean it will happen.

- Just because you've thought it doesn't mean it's the only way to think about it.

- What are alternative ways to think about it?

Attitudes and Actions that can help:

- If there's a problem, what are some options?

- Approach rather than avoid.

Results and Rewards:

- Set realistic expectations.

- Focus on efforts, not outcomes.

- Reinforce any approach of difficult situations with a reward.

Acknowledgements

We'd like to acknowledge the dedicated researchers and clinicians in the field of childhood anxiety and depression without whom this book could not have been written. The principles of CBT, our FEAR plan, and many of the suggested activities were developed over years and shaped by the writings and teachings of the outstanding friends, researchers and clinicians, Dr. Aaron T. Beck, Dr. John March, Dr. John Piacentini, Dr. Anne Marie Albano, Dr. Tamar Chansky, Dr. Martin Franklin, and Dr. Martin Seligman, among others. We'd also like to acknowledge Drs. Martha Kane, Bonnie Howard, Lynne Siqueland and Kristi Hedke who contributed to the emergence of the editions of The Coping Cat. Collectively, we thank you all, and the many others who worked with us along the way...and those whom we may have inadvertently omitted.

We are grateful to our esteemed friends and colleagues who reviewed and gave guidance and feedback along the way, Dr. Adam Grant, Dr. Eli Lebowitz, Dr. Anne Marie Albano, Darren Gold, Aneesh Chopra, Carl Eschenbach, Jen Morgan, Loren Danzis, and Laela Sturdy, thank you for inspiring our addition of "Conversation Starters."

Finally, to all the many children and families with whom we have worked over the years, thank you for sharing your lives with us, for taking on the challenges we presented, and for inspiring and teaching us along the way.

References

Barlow, David, Todd J. Farchione, Jacqueline R. Bullis, Matthew W. Gallagher, Heather Murray-Latin, Shannon Sauer-Zavala, Kate H. Bentley, et al. 2017. "The Unified Protocol for Transdiagnostic Treatment of Emotional Disorders Compared with Diagnosis-Specific Protocols for Anxiety Disorders: A Randomized Clinical Trial." *JAMA Psychiatry* 74 (9): 875–884.

Curran, T., & Hill, A. P. (2017). Perfectionism is increasing over time: A meta-analysis of birth cohort differences from 1989 to 2016. *Psychological Bulletin, 145*(4), 410–429.

Festinger, L. (1954). A theory of social comparison processes. *Human Relations, 7*(2), 117–140. https://doi.org/10.1177%2F001872675400700202

Flessner, C., Freeman, J. B., Sapyta, J., Garcia, A., Franklin, M.E., March, J. S., & Foa, E. (2011). Predictors of parental accommodation in pediatric obsessive-compulsive disorder: Findings from the Pediatric Obsessive-Compulsive Disorder Treatment Study (POTS) trial. *Journal of the American Academy of Child & Adolescent Psychiatry, 50,* 716–725.

Julian, K. (2020). What happened to American childhood? Too many kids show worrying signs of fragility from a very young age. Here's what we can do about it. *Atlantic* (May 2020). https://www.theatlantic.com/magazine/archive/2020/05/childhood-in-an-anxious-age/609079/

Kagan, E., Frank, H., & Kendall, P. C. (2017). Accommodation in youth with OCD and anxiety. *Clinical Psychology: Science and Practice, 24,* 78–98.

Kendall, Philip C. and Kristina Hedtke. 2006a. *Cognitive Behavioral Therapy for Anxious Children: Therapist Manual,* 3rd ed. Ardmore, PA: Workbook Publishing.

Kendall, Philip C. and Kristina Hedtke. 2006b. *Coping Cat Workbook,* 2nd ed. Ardmore, PA: Workbook Publishing.

Lebowitz, E. R., et al. (2013). Family accommodation in pediatric anxiety disorders. *Depression and Anxiety, 30,* 47–54.

Lebowitz, E. R., Scharfstein, L. A., & Jones, J. (2014). Comparing family accommodation in pediatric obsessive-compulsive disorder, anxiety disorders, and nonanxious children. *Depression and Anxiety, 31*(12), 1018–1025.

Montemayor, R. (1982). The relationship between parent-adolescent conflict and the amount of time adolescents spend alone and with parents and peers. *Child Development, 53*, 1512–1519. http://dx.doi.org/10.2307/1130078x

Peluso, M. A., & Guerra de Andrade, L. H. (2005). Physical activity and mental health: The association between exercise and mood. *Clinics, 60*(1), 61–70. doi:10.1590/s1807-59322005000100012

Peris, T., Bergman, R. L., Langley, A., Chang, S., McCracken, J., & Piacentini, J. (2008). Correlates of accommodation of pediatric obsessive-compulsive disorder: Parent, child, and family characteristics. *Journal of the American Academy of Child & Adolescent Psychiatry, 47*, 1173–1181.

Settipani, C., & Kendall, P. C. (2017). The effect of child distress on accommodation of anxiety: Relations with maternal beliefs, empathy, and anxiety. *Journal of Clinical Child and Adolescent Psychology, 46*, 810–823.

Smink, F. R., van Hoeken, D., & Hoek, H. W. (2012). Epidemiology of eating disorders: Incidence, prevalence, and mortality rates. *Current Psychiatry Reports, 14*(4), 406–14. doi:10.1007/s11920-012-0282-y. PMID: 22644309; PMCID: PMC3409365.

Thompson-Hollands, J., et al. (2014a). Family involvement in the psychological treatment of obsessive-compulsive disorder: A meta-analysis. *Journal of Family Psychology, 28*, 287–298.

Thompson-Hollands, J., et al. (2014b). Parental accommodation of child anxiety and related symptoms: Range, impact, and correlates. *Journal of Anxiety Disorders, 28*, 765–773.

Twenge, J., Joiner, T., Rogers, M., & Martin, G. (2017). Increases in depressive symptoms, suicide-related outcomes, and suicide rates among U.S. adolescents after 2010 and links to increased new media screen time. *Clinical Psychological Science, 6*(1), 216770261772337. doi:10.1177/2167702617723376.

Muniya S. Khanna, PhD, is a licensed clinical psychologist, and founder/director of The OCD & Anxiety Institute. Prior to this, Khanna served as faculty in the department of psychiatry at The University of Pennsylvania School of Medicine. She is an expert in the cognitive behavioral treatment of childhood anxiety and obsessive-compulsive spectrum disorders, having been involved in some of the most important research in the field in the last twenty years. Khanna is author of numerous scientific papers, chapters, and treatment manuals; and is a pioneer in web-based mental health research, spending the last decade working toward improving access to evidence-based mental health services in under-resourced populations by leveraging technology. In partnership with Philip C. Kendall, she developed digital interventions for child anxiety, including *Camp Cope-A-Lot* and *Child Anxiety Tales*; as well as hosting www.copingcatparents.com, a website to inform and empower parents of children and teens with anxiety.

Philip C. Kendall, PhD, ABPP, is a Distinguished University Professor and Laura H. Carnell professor of psychology at Temple University, where he is director of the Child and Adolescent Anxiety Disorders Clinic. He has produced more than 800 publications, including several books and more than twenty treatment manuals and workbooks. His treatment for anxiety in youth, *Coping Cat*, has been translated into over a dozen languages. *Coping Cat* has been evaluated in numerous randomized clinical trials conducted in different countries, examined by literature reviewers, and subsequently given the designation of an "empirically supported treatment." His contribution to our understanding and treatment of child anxiety is immeasurable.

Foreword writer **David H. Barlow, PhD**, is professor of psychology and psychiatry emeritus, and founder of the Center for Anxiety and Related Disorders at Boston University. He is past president of the Division of Clinical Psychology of the American Psychological Association, and past president of the Association for the Advancement of Behavior Therapy.

MORE BOOKS from
NEW HARBINGER PUBLICATIONS

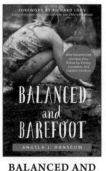
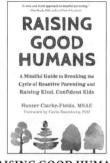
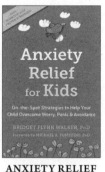
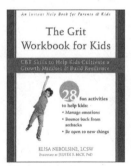
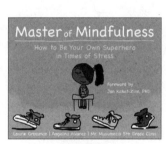
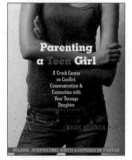

ABOUT US

Founded by psychologist Matthew McKay and Patrick
Fanning, New Harbinger has published books that
promote wellness in mind, body, and spirit for more than
forty-five years.

Our proven-effective self-help books and pioneering
workbooks help readers of all ages and backgrounds
make positive lifestyle changes, improve mental health
and well-being, and achieve meaningful personal growth.
In addition, our spirituality books offer profound
guidance for deepening awareness and cultivating
healing, self-discovery, and fulfillment.

New Harbinger is proud to be an independent and
employee-owned company, publishing books that reflect
its core values of integrity, innovation, commitment,
sustainability, compassion, and trust. Written by leaders
in the field and recommended by therapists worldwide,
New Harbinger books are practical, reliable, and provide
real tools for real change.

newharbingerpublications

Did you know there are free tools you can download for this book?

Free tools are things like **worksheets, guided meditation exercises**, and **more** that will help you get the most out of your book.

You can download free tools for this book—whether you bought or borrowed it, in any format, from any source— from the **New Harbinger** website. All you need is a NewHarbinger.com account. Just use the URL provided in this book to view the free tools that are available for it. Then, click on the "download" button for the free tool you want, and follow the prompts that appear to log in to your NewHarbinger.com account and download the material.

You can also save the free tools for this book to your **Free Tools Library** so you can access them again anytime, just by logging in to your account! Just look for this button on the book's free tools page:

+ save this to my
free tools library

If you need help accessing or downloading free tools, visit **newharbinger.com/faq** or contact us at customerservice@newharbinger.com.

CELEBRATING **40** YEARS